food *for* fitness

anita bean

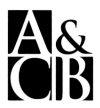

First published 1998 by

A & C Black Publishers Ltd
38 Soho Square, London W1D 3HB
www.acblack.com

Second edition 2002
Reprinted 1999, 2001
Copyright © 1998, 2002, 2007

ISBN-10: 0 7136 8128 4
ISBN-13: 978 0 7136 8128 4

The right of Anita Bean to be identified as the author of this work has been asserted by her in accordance with the Copyright, Designs and Patents Act 1988.

A CIP catalogue record for this book is available from the British Library.

Note: It is always the responsibility of the individual to assess his or her own fitness capability before participating in any training activity. Whilst every effort has been made to ensure the content of this book is as technically accurate as possible, neither the author nor the publishers can accept responsibility for any injury or loss sustained as a result of the use of this material.

Text and cover design by James Watson
Cover photograph of women eating bowl of cereal courtesy of © Getty Images (Adam Gault)
All other cover photographs courtesy of © Bananastock

This book is produced using paper that is made from wood grown in managed, sustainable forests. It is natural, renewable and recyclable. The logging and manufacturing processes conform to the environmental regulations of the country of origin.

Typeset in Norfolk by Fakenham Photosettting
Printed and bound in China by C & C Offset Printing Co., Ltd.

contents

introduction

When I visit gyms and sports clubs or speak to people who workout regularly I am constantly bombarded by questions about what to eat. The most frequently asked questions are what to eat before, during and after training; how to lose weight without losing energy; how much to drink; and which sports supplements work. It's great that so many of you care about your diet but it's also very clear to me that there is a lot of misinformation out there.

That's why I've written this book. The intention is to give you accurate, practical and easy-to-follow guidance about what to eat for peak performance. I've included the most up-to-date science on the subject and attempted to answer all your questions as honestly as possible.

To help you put the advice in this book into practice, I developed 99 recipes for you to try. I wanted to help you share in the enjoyment of good food and healthy eating and inspire you to get cooking. All the dishes are easy and quick to prepare – advanced cooking skills are definitely not required! All of the recipes can be prepared in less than thirty minutes.

The recipes are simple and can be easily sourced from any supermarket (as well as local markets and corner shops). There's no need to buy anything from specialist shops. The main thing is to choose the freshest and best-quality foods you can find. Buy seasonal and locally grown produce if you can. Try to shop little and often for fresh produce so you get the most goodness from it.

This book is a nutrition guide, a practical handbook and a recipe book all rolled into one. I hope that it helps you take your workouts to the next level.

Enjoy!

Anita

acknowledgements

There are a number of people I would like to thank: my husband Simon for his balanced perspective on life and his patience with my late nights; my beautiful daughters Chloe and Lucy for their love of life and giving me inspiration to write; Rob Foss and Lucy Beevor at A & C Black for their editorial expertise and for making this book possible; and finally all the athletes with whom I have worked over the years for sharing their experience with me.

foreword

I am a great believer in an active lifestyle. I know from first-hand experience that diet plays a very big part in any fitness programme as well as sporting success. When I was training for the Olympics, I would eat a lot of food – a typical week would include more than twenty hours in the pool as well as ten in the gym – so I was always hungry. But, to be the best in my sport, I made sure that I ate a lot of the right foods, as well as trained very hard. I won an Olympic silver medal, double Commonwealth gold, competed in three Olympics in three decades, as well as set 200 British records. I now work for the BBC as a presenter on swimming, amongst other things.

Although I no longer compete, I am still committed to a fitness regime. These days I basically exercise to stay in shape – regularly working out in my home gym, skiing, walking the dog and playing with my kids – but I still pay attention to what I eat. I don't diet, I've tried them, and they don't work for me. I just eat healthily, balancing what I eat with my activity needs. When I eat well, I have more energy and I perform a lot better, too. It's simple really, calories in equals calories out – or you start to put on more weight!

I've known Anita for several years and always shared her practical approach to nutrition. I welcome this book – it combines the best of nutrition knowledge with fitness training and an active lifestyle. It gives you clear no-nonsense advice about what to eat, how much to eat and when to eat. There are hundreds of useful facts and tips to help you put together a healthy eating plan, whether you are working out for fitness or in serious training for competitions. I'm sure that you will find this book useful and a great investment in your well-being.

Sharron Davies MBE Olympic Swimming Champion

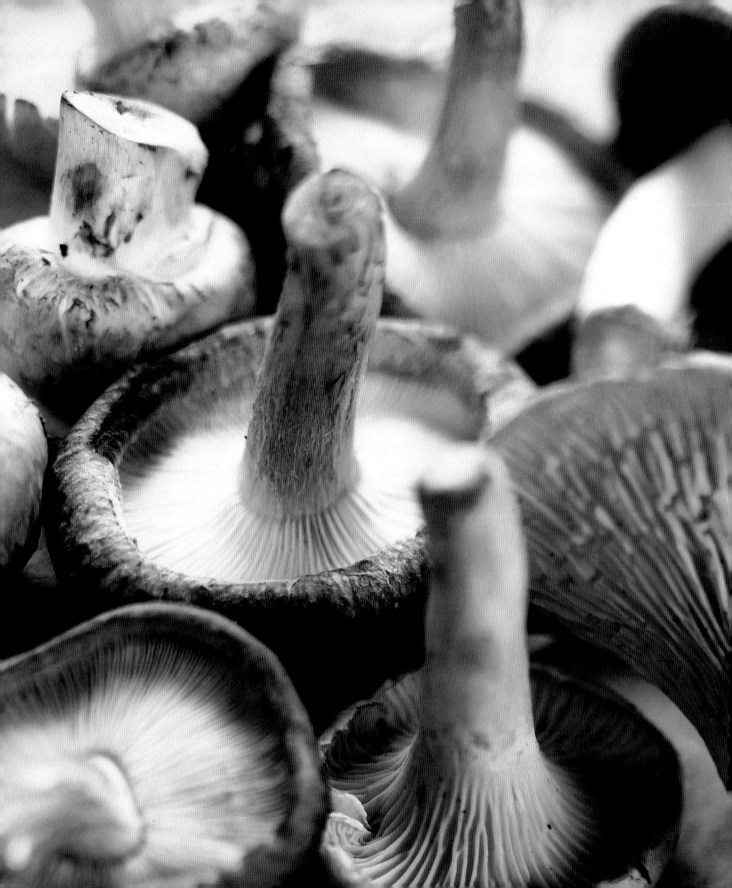

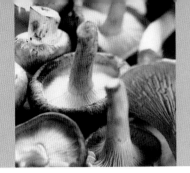

1 nutrition guide

Regular exercise taxes every cell and every system in your body: your muscles, joints, ligaments, tendons, respiratory, circulatory and immune systems all have to work harder when you exercise. Eating a healthy diet can help minimise the damage caused by exercise and help your body rebuild itself even stronger.

Your daily diet needs to meet the tough demands of your training programme as well as keep you healthy. To help you make the right food choices, this chapter explains the basis of a good training diet, what each nutrient does, how much you need and how you can achieve your ideal intake.

1. Energy (calories)

Where do I get energy?

You get energy from four components in food and drink: carbohydrate, fat, protein and alcohol. These fuels are broken down in your body and transformed via various biochemical pathways into a compound called adenosine triphosphate (ATP). Energy is produced when one of the phosphate molecules splits off, leaving adenosine diphosphate (ADP). This energy can then be used to fuel your muscles.

weigh it up

Each nutrient provides different amounts of energy. 1 g provides:

alcohol	7 kcal (29 kJ)
carbohydrate	4 kcal (17 kJ)
fat	9 kcal (38 kJ)
protein	4 kcal (17 kJ)

CALORIES EXPLAINED

One calorie is the amount of heat required to increase the temperature of 1 gram of water by 1 °C. But, as this is a very small amount of energy, we mostly work with larger units called kilocalories (kcal), which is 1,000 calories. You have probably seen these units on food labels. When we mention calories in the everyday sense, we are really talking about kilocalories.

You'll also see food energy measured in joules or kilojoules on food labels, which is the SI (International Unit System) unit for energy. One Joule is the work required to exert a force of 1 Newton for a distance of 1 metre. One kcal is equivalent to 4.2 kJ, so to convert kilocalories into kilojoules, multiply by 4.2. To convert kilojoules into kilocalories, divide by 4.2.

How many calories do I need?

You can estimate your daily calorie needs by working out your basal metabolic rate (BMR) and multiplying it by your physical activity level.

Your BMR is the number of calories you burn at rest over 24 hours maintaining essential functions such as respiration, digestion and brain function. BMR accounts for 60–75 per cent of the calories you burn daily.

Step 1: Estimate your basal metabolic rate (BMR):

(A) Quick method: As a rule of thumb, BMR uses 11 calories for every 0.5 kg of a woman's body weight and 12 calories per 0.5 kg of a man's body weight.

Women: BMR = weight in kilos × 2 × 11 (alternatively weight in pounds × 11)

Men: BMR = weight in kilos × 2 × 12 (alternatively weight in pounds × 12)

Example: BMR for a 60 kg woman = 60 × 2 × 11 = 1,320 kcal.

(B) Longer method: For a more accurate estimation of your BMR, use the following equations:

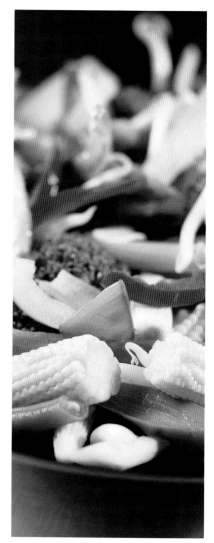

Age	Men	Women
10–18 years	(weight in kg × 17.5) + 651	(weight in kg × 12.2) + 746
18–30 years	(weight in kg × 15.3) + 679	(weight in kg × 14.7) + 479
31–60 years	(weight in kg × 11.6) + 879	(weight in kg × 8.7) + 829
60+ years	(weight in kg × 13.5) + 487	(weight in kg × 10.5) + 596

Example: BMR for a 60 kg woman aged 31–60 years = (60 × 8.7) + 829 = 1,351 kcal.

Step 2: Estimate your physical activity level (PAL):

Your physical activity level (PAL) is the ratio of your overall daily energy expenditure to your BMR. It's a rough measure of your lifestyle activity.

Mostly inactive or sedentary (mainly sitting): 1.2
Fairly active (include walking and exercise 1–2 × week): 1.3
Moderately active (exercise 2–3 × weekly): 1.4
Active (exercise hard more than 3 × weekly): 1.5
Very active (exercise hard daily): 1.7

Step 3: Multiply your BMR by your PAL to work out your daily calorie needs:

BMR × PAL

Example: daily energy needs for an active 60 kg woman = 1,351 × 1.5 = 2,027 kcal.

That's how many calories you burn a day to maintain your weight, assuming you have an 'average' body composition. If you have higher than average muscle mass add 150 calories.

To lose weight, reduce your daily calorie intake by 15 per cent or multiply the figure above (maintenance calorie needs) by 0.85. This will produce a fat loss of about 0.5 kg per week.

Example: Daily energy needs for an active 60 kg woman to lose weight = 2,027 × 0.85 = 1,723 kcal.

To gain weight, increase your daily calorie intake by 20 per cent or multiply the figure above (maintenance calorie needs) by 1.2. In conjunction with a resistance training programme, expect a weight gain of 0.25–0.5 kg per month.

Example: Daily energy needs for an active 60 kg woman to gain weight = 2,027 × 1.2 = 2,432 kcal.

2. Carbohydrate

Why do you need carbohydrate?

Carbohydrate is your main source of energy. Your brain, nervous system and heart need a constant supply of carbohydrate (in the form of blood glucose) in order to function properly. You also need carbohydrate to fuel your muscles.

The carbohydrates in your food are converted into glycogen and stored in your muscles. Rather like filling your car up with petrol before a journey, you need to ensure your muscles are well fuelled before working out.

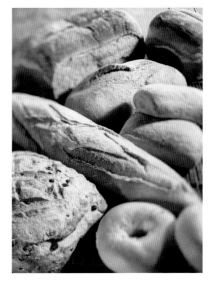

How much?

The more active you are, the more carbohydrate you need to fuel your muscles. Regular exercisers training up to 2 hours daily need around 4–7 g of carbohydrate for each kg of their body weight, or approximately 50–60 per cent of their total calorie intake. Serious athletes who train 4 hours or more a day may need as much as 10 g.

The box below provides a guide to your carbohydrate needs, based on body weight and activity level. For example, if you weigh 70 kg and work out 3–5 hours a week, you'll need 4–5 g per kg a day, or between (70 × 4) and (70 × 5) = 280–350 g carbohydrate daily.

HOW MUCH CARBOHYDRATE?	
Activity level	**g/oz. carbohydrate per day**
3–5 hours per week	4–5 g
5–7 hours per week	5–6 g
1–2 hours per day	6–7 g
2–4 hours per day	7–8 g
More than 4 hours per day	8–10 g

Simple or complex?

Carbohydrates are traditionally classified as simple (mono- or disaccharides) or complex (polysaccharides) according to the number of sugar units in the molecules. But this tells you very little about their effect on your body and your blood glucose level. Today, carbohydrates are more commonly categorised according to their glycaemic index (GI).

What's the GI?

The GI is a measure of how the body reacts to foods containing carbohydrate. To make a fair comparison, all foods are compared with a reference food, normally glucose, and are tested in equivalent carbohydrate amounts. Glucose has a GI score of 100.

How does GI affect the body?

High GI foods cause a rapid rise in blood glucose levels and have a GI number above 70 (glucose has the highest score at 100). They include refined starchy foods such as potatoes, cornflakes, white bread and white rice as well as sugary foods such as soft drinks, biscuits and sweets.

TOO LITTLE OR TOO MUCH CARBOHYDRATE?

A good guide to whether you are eating enough carbohydrate is how energetic you feel during your workouts. If you feel easily fatigued, this suggests low glycogen levels and an insufficient carbohydrate intake. Upping your carbohydrate intake by an extra 50–100 g daily should boost energy levels and stave off fatigue. However, over-eating carbohydrates won't increase your energy levels. Instead, you may feel 'heavy' and, ironically, more lethargic. Once your glycogen stores are filled, excess carbohydrates are converted into fat so you may notice that you put on weight. Try to listen to your body and you'll soon find the balance between too little and too much carbohydrate.

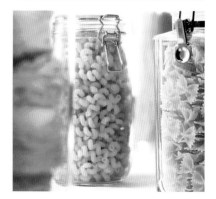

Foods classed as low GI fall below 55 and produce a slower and smaller rise in blood glucose levels. They include beans, lentils, coarse grain breads, muesli, fruit and dairy products. Moderate GI foods such as porridge, rice and sweet potatoes have a GI between 55 and 70.

Protein-rich foods such as meat, fish, chicken and eggs and pure fats such as oils, butter and margarine contain no carbohydrate so these foods have no GI value. But adding these foods – as well as fats and low GI carbohydrate foods – to meals will reduce the GI of the entire meal. Cooking and ripening (of fruits) tends to increase the GI value.

See page 7 for an easy guide to foods with a high, moderate and low GI.

Low GI eating at a glance

Essentially, a low GI diet comprises carbohydrate foods with a low GI as well as lean protein foods and healthy fats. Low GI foods include:

Fresh fruit

The more acidic the fruit, the lower the GI. Apples, pears, oranges, grapefruit, peaches, nectarines, plums and apricots have the lowest GI values while tropical fruits such as pineapple, papaya and watermelon have higher values. However, as average portion size is small, the GL (*see* page 7) would be low.

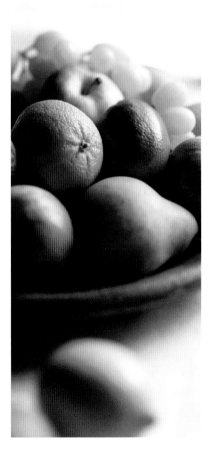

Fresh vegetables

Most vegetables have a very low carbohydrate content and don't have a GI value (you would need to eat enormous amounts to get a significant rise in blood glucose). The exception is potatoes, which have a high GI. Eat them with protein/or healthy fat or replace with low GI starchy vegetables.

Low GI starchy vegetables

These include sweetcorn (GI 46–48), sweet potato (GI 46), and yam (GI 37).

Low GI breads

These include stone-ground wholemeal bread (not ordinary wholemeal bread), fruit or malt loaf, wholegrain bread with lots of grainy bits, breads containing barley, rye, oats, soy and cracked wheat or those containing sunflower seeds or linseeds, chapatti and pitta breads (unleavened), pumpernickel (rye kernel) bread, and sourdough bread.

Low GI breakfast cereals

These include porridge, muesli and other oat or rye-based cereals, and high bran cereals (e.g. All Bran).

Low GI grains

These include bulgar wheat, noodles, oats, pasta, basmati rice (not ordinary brown or white rice).

Beans and lentils

These include chickpeas, red kidney beans, baked beans, cannelloni beans, mung beans, black-eyed beans, butter beans, split peas and lentils.

Nuts and seeds

Nuts include almonds, brazils, cashews, hazelnuts, pine nuts, pistachios, and peanuts. Seeds include sunflower, sesame, flax and pumpkin seeds.

Fish, lean meat, poultry and eggs

These contain no carbohydrate and so have no GI value.

Low-fat dairy products

Milk, cheese and yoghurt are important for their calcium and protein content. Opt for lower fat versions where possible.

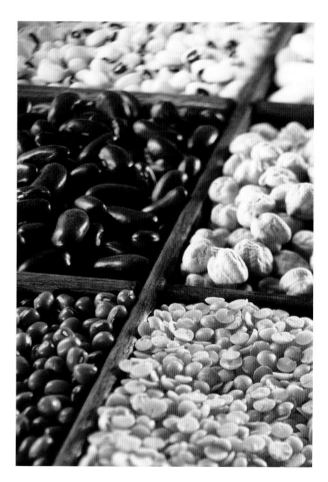

AN EASY GI GUIDE

Low GI foods	Moderate GI foods	High GI foods
Sweetcorn	Pineapple	White bread and rolls, French bread, bagels
Sweet potato and yam	Raisins and sultanas	Regular sliced wholemeal bread
Most vegetables, e.g. cucumber, broccoli	Oatcakes and rye crispbread	Most breakfast cereals, e.g. cornflakes, rice crispies, bran flakes
Most fresh fruit, e.g. apples, pears, oranges, peaches, apricots, bananas, grapes, kiwi fruit, strawberries, mangoes	Wholegrain (brown) and basmati rice	Breakfast bars
	Dried figs	Crackers and rice cakes
Beans, chickpeas and lentils	Chapatti	White rice
Low fat dairy products, e.g. milk and yoghurt, soya 'milk'	Pitta bread	Gluten-free bread and pasta
	Rice noodles	Mashed, boiled and baked potatoes
Pasta	Jam	Doughnuts
Rye bread, coarse grain bread, stone-ground wholemeal bread, breads containing oats, soy, cracked wheat, or seeds	Tinned fruit	Chips
	Ice cream	Sugar
Bulgur wheat, cous cous, barley*	Raisins	Soft drinks
Fish, poultry and lean meat	Muesli bars	Sweets
Most fruit juice	Digestive biscuits	Most biscuits
Nuts and seeds		
Porridge, oatmeal, and muesli		
Honey		

What is the glycaemic load?

The glycaemic load (GL) gives you a more accurate idea of how a food behaves in your body. Unlike GI, it takes account of the portion size (that is, the amount of carbohydrate you are eating) so can be regarded as a measure of both the quantity and quality of the carbohydrate.

It is calculated as follows:

GL = (GI × carbohydrate per portion) ÷ 100

One unit of GL is roughly equivalent to the glycaemic effect of 1 g of glucose.

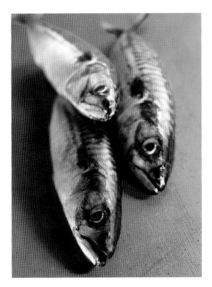

So, for watermelon:

GL = (72 × 6) ÷ 100 = 4.3

	GI value	GL value	Daily GL total
Low	0–55	0–10	0–80
Medium	56–70	11–19	80–120
High	71–100	> 20	> 120

For optimal glycogen storage and minimal fat storage, aim to achieve a small or moderate glycaemic load – eat little and often, avoid overloading on carbohydrates, and stick to balanced combinations of carbohydrate, protein and healthy fat.

Which is best – GI or GL?

A major problem with the GI is that it doesn't take account of portion size, and so it can create a falsely bad impression of a food. For example, watermelon with a GI of 72 – classified as a high-GI food – is off the menu on a low-GI diet. However, an average slice (120 g/4.2 oz.) provides only 6 g carbohydrate, not enough to significantly raise your blood glucose level. You would need to eat 720 g of watermelon to obtain 50 g carbohydrate – the amount used in the GI test.

Another drawback is that some high-fat foods have a low GI, which gives a falsely favourable impression of the food. For example, crisps have a lower GI (54) than baked potatoes (85). But they are easy to overeat because they are high in fat (often saturated fat) and are calorie-dense, but not very filling. Don't select foods only by their GI – check the type of fat (i.e. saturated or unsaturated) and avoid those that contain large amounts of saturated or trans fats.

Q&A

Question: *"I've been trying to lose weight by following a low-GI diet. I've heard that low-GI foods should keep me feeling fuller for longer but they don't, nor am I losing weight."*

Answer: Foods with a low GI are generally more nutritious than higher-GI foods, but to lose weight you still have to consume fewer calories than you burn. In theory, a low-GI diet should be filling and satisfying because many foods with a low-GI are high in fibre and take longer to digest, so helping to curb your appetite. In practice, it's quite easy to unwittingly load up on calories. Muesli (GI 49), boiled potatoes (GI 50), spaghetti (GI 48) and sponge cake (GI 46) are all low-GI foods but are also relatively high in calories. Even milk chocolate has a respectable GI (43) but provides as many as 240 calories (1,004 kJ) per 45 g bar!

There have been no long-term studies, but of the short-term studies to date only about half have found that low-GI foods reduce hunger, increase satiety (feelings of fullness) or reduce overall food intake. No difference in satiety or food intake was found in the remaining half. A study published in the *American Journal of Clinical Nutrition* in 2004 found that weight loss on a low-GI diet was no different to that on a high-GI diet.

Clearly, a low-GI value isn't a license to eat freely; you still have to keep a reign on portion sizes. To lose weight eat higher-calorie or carb-dense low-GI foods in moderation (cereals, breads, grains, full-fat dairy products, desserts, confectionery and bakery items) only and fill up instead on fibre-rich low-GI foods with a high water content (fresh fruits, vegetables, salads).

EAT LIKE AN ATHLETE

Studies at the University of Sydney, Australia, have found that athletes produce much less insulin than the GI index suggests after eating high-GI foods. In other words, athletes don't show the same peaks and troughs in blood glucose and insulin as sedentary people do. But this doesn't give athletes a licence to pig out on high-GI foods. They should regard the GI index as a guide to show how various foods are likely to behave in the body.

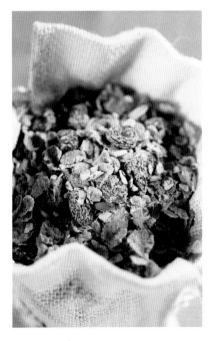

3. Fibre

What is it?

Fibre is the term used to describe the complex carbohydrates found in plants that are resistant to digestion. There are two kinds of fibre – insoluble and soluble. Most plant foods contain both, but proportions vary. Good sources of insoluble fibre include wholewheat bread and other wheat products, brown rice and vegetables. These help to speed the passage of food through your gut, and prevent constipation and bowel problems. Soluble fibre, found in pulses, fruit and vegetables, reduces 'bad' LDL cholesterol levels and helps control blood glucose levels by slowing glucose absorption. High-fibre foods are beneficial for weight loss as they fill you up and help to satisfy your appetite.

How much?

The Department of Health recommends between 18 g and 24 g a day, although for people prone to constipation up to 32 g a day would be advisable. The average intake in the United Kingdom is around 13 g a day.

4. Protein

Why do you need protein?

Protein is needed for the growth, formation and repair of body cells. It is also needed for making enzymes, hormones and antibodies.

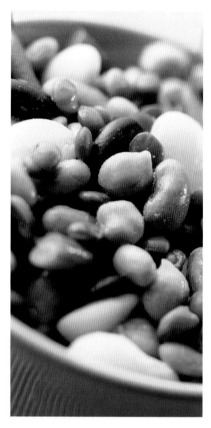

How much?

The Recommended Daily Amount (RDA – *see page 18*) for the general population is 0.75 g per kg of body weight a day. For example, for a 70 kg person the amount should be 53 g.

Regular exercisers need more protein than inactive people to compensate for the increased muscle breakdown that occurs during and after intense exercise, as well as to build new muscle cells. You'll need between 1.2 and 1.8 g of protein per kg of bodyweight daily, depending on your sport and how hard you workout. If you do mostly endurance activities, such as running, aim to consume 1.2–1.4 g protein per kg (2.2 lb.) bodyweight a day. That's 84–98 g daily for a 70 kg person. If you include regular strength and power activities, such as weight training, in your programme aim for 1.4–1.8 g per kg (2.2 lb.) of bodyweight a day. This is 98–126 g daily – approximately 20–25 per cent of your calorie intake. Skimping on protein can cause fatigue and slow recovery after workouts. It will result in slower muscle and strength gains.

See page 11 for the protein content of various foods.

THE PROTEIN CONTENT OF VARIOUS FOODS

Food	Protein (g)
Meat and fish	
1 lean fillet steak (105 g)	31 g
1 chicken breast fillet (125 g)	30 g
2 slices turkey breast (40 g)	10 g
1 salmon fillet (150 g)	30 g
Tuna, canned in brine	24 g
Dairy products	
1 slice (40 g) Cheddar cheese	10 g
2 tablespoons (112 g) cottage cheese	15 g
1 glass (200 ml) skimmed milk	7 g
1 glass (200 ml) soya milk	7 g
1 carton yoghurt (150 g)	6 g
1 egg (size 2)	8 g
Nuts and seeds	
1 handful (50 g) peanuts	12 g
1 tablespoon (20 g) peanut butter	5 g
Pulses	
1 small tin (205 g) baked beans	10 g
3 tablespoons (120 g) cooked lentils	9 g
3 tablespoons (120 g) cooked red kidney beans	10 g
Soya and quorn products	
1 tofu burger (60 g)	5 g
1 quorn burger (50 g)	6 g
Grains and cereals	
2 slices wholemeal bread	6 g
1 serving (230 g) cooked pasta	7 g
Protein supplements	
1 scoop (32 g) protein powder	22 g *
1 serving (76 g) meal replacement shake	42 g *
1 nutrition (sports) bar (50 g)	15 g *

* Values may vary depending on brand

Best sources?

You should get the majority of your protein from food sources rather than supplements. Animal sources such as poultry, fish, meat, dairy products and eggs generally have a higher biological value (BV) (*see* 'Protein fact file' on page 33) than plant sources such as tofu, quorn, beans, lentils, nuts and cereals.

AMINO ACIDS EXPLAINED

Amino acids are the small components of protein. They are often called the building blocks of the body because they are used to repair muscle tissue. Eight amino acids must be provided by the diet (the 'essential amino acids'), while the body produces the others.

All eight essential amino acids have to be present for your body to use food proteins properly. Animal proteins, as well as soya and quorn, contain a good balance of the essential amino acids. However, plant proteins such as pulses, cereals and nuts contain smaller amounts. The general rule is to combine plant proteins to make a full complement of amino acids (e.g. beans on toast, lentils and rice, peanut butter on bread).

If you eat a mixture of animal and plant sources, you will get a good balance of amino acids as well as a wider range of other nutrients such as fibre, vitamins, minerals and carbohydrate. To minimise your fat intake, opt for lean protein sources like skinless poultry, low fat dairy products and pulses.

5. Fat

Why do you need fat?

Fat is part of the structure of every membrane of every cell in your body. Fat also provides essential fatty acids (*see* pages 15–17), vitamins A, D and E, and is a concentrated source of energy, providing 9 calories per gram. Aim for most of your fat to be the 'good' unsaturated kind while avoiding 'bad' saturated and trans fats.

How much?

Sports science researchers recommend regular exercisers consume 20–25 per cent of calories from fat (The American Dietetic Association and ACSM, 2000). This is in line with the maximum recommended for the general population by the World Health Organisation (less than 30 per cent of calories) and the UK Department of Health (less than 33 per cent of calories), but less than the current average intake of the general population (35–36 per cent).

Using the ACSM recommendations, regular exercisers eating 2,500 kcal (10,460 kJ) a day should aim for 56–69 g of fat. This is lower than the Guideline Daily Amount (GDA) for fat recommended to the general population by the UK Food Standards Agency (FSA): 95 g for men and 70 g for women.

Bad fats

Saturated fats are found in animal fats and products made with palm oil or palm kernel oil. They raise blood cholesterol levels and increase the risk of heart disease, so they have no beneficial role in keeping the body healthy. Recognising that it would be impractical to cut saturated fats out altogether, the UK Department of Health recommends that no more than 10 per cent of total calories come from saturated fat. The GDA is 30 g for men and 20 g for women.

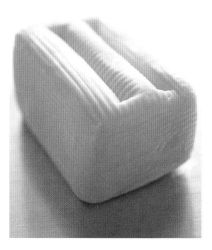

Main sources include:

- Fatty meats
- Full-fat dairy products
- Butter
- Lard, shortening, dripping
- Palm oil ('vegetable fat')
- Palm kernel oil ('vegetable fat')
- Margarine, spreads, biscuits, cakes, desserts, etc made with palm or palm kernel oil
- Egg yolk

Trans fats are even more harmful than saturated fats. Tiny amounts occur naturally in meat and dairy products, but most are formed artificially during the commercial process of hydrogenation when vegetable oils are converted into hardened *hydrogenated fats*. Hard fats are a cheap way to make pastries and biscuits crispy, cakes moist and fillings creamy, and many processed foods last longer. But they increase blood levels of LDL cholesterol ('bad' cholesterol) while lowering HDL ('good') cholesterol, which increases your risk of heart disease. They may also encourage fat deposition around your middle, according to a 2006 US study, and increase the risk of diabetes.

There is no level of trans fatty acids that is safe, according to the US Institute of Medicine, who recommends that we should aim for zero. The UK Department of Health recommends that trans fatty acids make up no more than 2 per cent of total calorie intake – roughly 5 g per day. Check food labels for hydrogenated fats and *partially hydrogenated fats*.

Main sources include:

- Margarine
- Low-fat spread
- Pastries, pies and tarts
- Biscuits

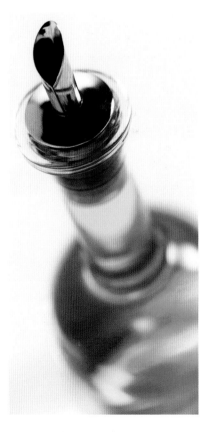

- Cereal bars, breakfast bars
- Cakes and bakery products
- Crackers
- Ice cream
- Desserts and puddings
- Fried food

Good fats

Monounsaturated fats lower harmful LDL cholesterol levels (without affecting 'good' HDL) and can cut your heart disease and cancer risk. The Department of Health recommends an intake of up to 12 per cent of total calories.

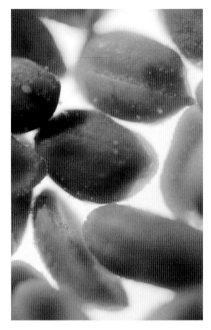

Main sources include:

- Olive oil, olive oil margarine
- Rapeseed oil
- Avocados
- Soya oil
- Peanuts, almonds, cashews
- Peanut butter
- Sunflower and sesame seeds
- Mayonnaise

Polyunsaturated fats in moderation also reduce the risk of heart disease, though less effectively than monounsaturated fats. The Department of Health recommends a maximum intake of 10 per cent of total calories. Two types of polyunsaturated fats – the omega-3 and omega-6 fatty acids – are extremely important for maintaining the correct structure of cell membranes in the body.

Main sources include:

- Sunflower oil
- Corn oil

■ Safflower oil

■ Sunflower oil margarine

■ Nuts and seeds

Omega-3 fatty acids include the short-chain fatty acid alpha linolenic acid (found in plant sources), and the long-chain fatty acids eicosapentanoic acid (EPA) and docosahexanoic acid (DHA), both found only in fish oils. They are necessary for proper functioning of the brain, regulating hormones, for the immune system and blood flow. Omega-3 fatty acids protect against heart disease and stroke and, according to recent research, may also help improve brain function, prevent Alzheimer's disease, treat depression, and help improve the behaviour of children with dyslexia, dyspraxia and ADHD. For regular exercisers, omega-3s increase the delivery of oxygen to muscles, and improve aerobic capacity and endurance. They also help to speed-up recovery and reduce inflammation and joint stiffness.

You only need small amounts of omega-3 fatty acids to keep you healthy. But, as they are found in relatively few foods, many people struggle to meet the minimum requirement of 0.9 g a day. Aim to eat a minimum 140 g portion of oily fish a week or one tablespoon of an omega-3 rich oil daily. The omega-3 content of various foods is shown on page 17.

Main sources include:

■ Sardines

■ Mackerel

■ Salmon

■ Fresh (not tinned) tuna

■ Trout

■ Herring

■ Walnuts

■ Walnut oil

■ Pumpkin seeds

■ Pumpkinseed oil

- Flaxseeds
- Flaxseed oil
- Rapeseed oil
- Soya oil
- Sweet potatoes
- Omega-3 enriched eggs, bread, margarine and fruit juice

Omega-6 fatty acids include linolenic acid and gamma linolenic acid (GLA) and are easier to find in foods than omega-3s. For this reason, most people currently eat too much omega-6 in relation to omega-3, which results in an imbalance of prostaglandins ('mini' hormone responsible for controlling blood clotting, inflammation and the immune system). The average diet contains a ratio of 10:1. Aim for a ratio of no more than five times the amount of omega-6s as omega-3s.

Main sources include:

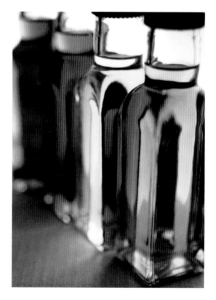

- Sunflower oil
- Sunflower oil margarine
- Safflower oil
- Corn oil
- Groundnut oil
- Olive oil
- Peanuts
- Peanut butter
- Evening primrose oil
- Sunflower and sesame seeds

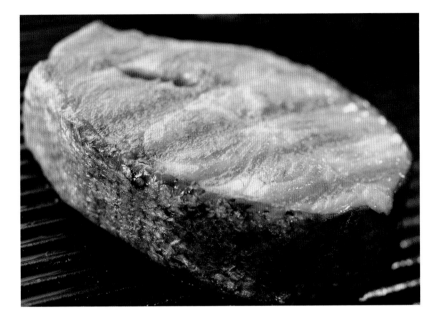

SOURCES OF OMEGA-3 FATTY ACIDS

Food	Omega-3 fatty acids: g per 100 g	Portion size	Omega-3 fatty acids: g per portion
Salmon	2.5 g	100 g	2.5 g
Mackerel	2.8 g	160 g	4.5 g
Sardines (tinned)	2.0 g	100 g	2.0 g
Trout	1.3 g	230 g	2.9 g
Tuna (canned in oil, drained)	1.1 g	100 g	1.1 g
Cod liver oil	24 g	1 tsp (5 ml)	1.2 g
Flaxseed oil	57 g	1 tbsp (14 ml)	8.0 g
Flaxseeds (ground)	16 g	1 tbsp (24 g)	3.8 g
Rapeseed oil	9.6 g	1 tbsp (14 ml)	1.3 g
Walnuts	7.5 g	1 tbsp (28 g)	2.6 g
Walnut oil	11.5 g	1 tbsp (14 ml)	1.6 g
Sweet potatoes	0.03 g	Medium (130 g)	1.3 g
Peanuts	0.4 g	Handful (50 g)	0.2 g
Broccoli	0.1 g	3 tbsp (125 g)	1.3 g
Pumpkin seeds	8.5 g	2 tbsp (25 g)	2.1 g
Omega-3 eggs		1 egg	0.7 g
Typical omega-3 supplement		8 capsules	0.5 g

6. Vitamins and Minerals

Why do you need them?

Vitamins and minerals are substances that are needed in tiny amounts to enable your body to work properly and prevent illness. Getting the right balance of vitamins and minerals will also help your sports performance.

Vitamins support the immune system, help the brain function properly and aid the conversion of food into energy. They are important for healthy skin and hair, controlling growth and balancing hormones. The B vitamins and vitamin C must be provided daily by the diet, as they cannot be stored.

Minerals are needed for structural and regulatory functions, including bone strength, haemoglobin manufacture, fluid balance and muscle contraction.

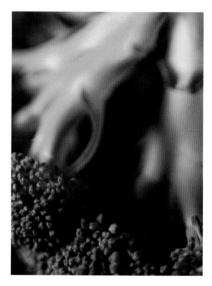

How much?

The Essential Guide to Vitamins and Minerals on pages 19–21 summarises the exercise-related functions, best food sources, and requirements of twelve key vitamins and minerals. But regular exercise places additional demands on your body, and your RDA for many vitamins and minerals is likely to be higher than the RDAs for the general population. Failure to meet your RDAs may leave you lacking in energy and susceptible to minor infections and illnesses.

ARE YOU DEFICIENT IN VITAMINS AND MINERALS?

A study published in the *Journal of the American Medical Association* concluded that most people do not get enough vitamins in their diet to protect themselves from diseases such as cancer and heart disease. Researchers at the Harvard Medical School say that most people would benefit from taking a multivitamin, especially if:

- ■ You are dieting or eating fewer than 1,500 calories (6,276 kJ) daily. Restricting your food intake means you are likely to miss out on certain nutrients.

- ■ You rely mainly on processed or fast foods, which are high in saturated fat, sugar and salt, and depleted in vitamins.

WHAT ARE RDAS?

The Recommended Daily Amounts (RDAs) listed on food and supplement labels are estimates of nutrient requirements set by the EU and designed to cover the needs of the majority of a population. The amounts are intended to prevent deficiency symptoms, allow for a little storage, as well as covering differences in needs from one person to the next. They are not targets; rather they are guides to help you check that your body is getting enough nutrients.

ARE YOU DEFICIENT IN VITAMINS AND MINERALS? (CONTINUED)

- You regularly skip meals, and therefore you are more likely to eat high-calorie snacks that are low in vitamins and minerals.

- You don't eat the recommended five portions of fruit and vegetable daily. These foods are rich in vitamins, minerals and antioxidants.

- You have a food intolerance or allergy. It may be harder to get some of the nutrients you need.

- You are a vegan. It's more difficult (though not impossible) to get enough vitamin B12, calcium and iron from a plant-based diet.

- You are pregnant. Take a supplement containing 0.4 mg of folic acid and follow the advice of your midwife or doctor.

About 12 million people in the UK take vitamin and mineral supplements to prevent or alleviate illnesses.

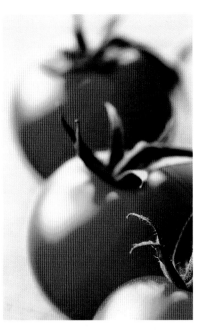

ESSENTIAL GUIDE TO VITAMINS AND MINERALS

Vitamin/mineral	How much? *	Why is it needed?	Benefits	Best food sources	Side effects
Vitamin A	700 µg (men) 600 mg (women) No SUL ** FSA recommends 1500 µg max	Helps vision in dim light; promotes healthy skin	Helps to maintain normal vision and healthy skin	Liver, cheese, oily fish, eggs, butter, margarine	Liver and bone damage; may cause birth defects (avoid during pregnancy)
Carotenoids (also act as antioxidants)	No official RNI 15 mg beta-carotene suggested SUL = 7 mg beta-carotene	Vision in dim light; healthy skin; converts into vitamin A	May protect against certain cancers; may reduce muscle soreness. (Exercise increases need for antioxidants.)	Intensely coloured fruit and vegetables, e.g. apricots, peppers, tomatoes, mangoes, broccoli	Excessive doses of beta-carotene can cause harmless orange tinge to skin. Reversible.
Thiamin	0.4 mg/ 1,000 kcal No SUL FSA recommends 100 mg max	Converts carbohydrates to energy	Processes extra carbohydrate consumed	Wholemeal bread and cereals, pulses, meat	Excess is excreted so toxicity is rare
Riboflavin	1.3 mg (men) 1.1 mg (women) No SUL FSA recommends 40 mg max	Converts carbohydrates to energy	Processes extra carbohydrate consumed	Milk and dairy products, meat, eggs	Excess is excreted (producing yellow urine) so toxicity is rare

ESSENTIAL GUIDE TO VITAMINS AND MINERALS (CONTINUED)

Vitamin/mineral	How much? *	Why is it needed?	Benefits	Best food sources	Side effects
Niacin	6.6 mg/ 1,000 kcal SUL = 17 mg	Converts carbohydrates to energy	Processes the extra carbohydrate consumed	Meat and offal, nuts, milk and dairy products, eggs, wholegrain cereals	Excess is excreted. High doses may cause hot flushes
Vitamin C	40 mg SUL = 1,000 mg	Healthy connective tissue, bones, teeth, blood vessels, gums and teeth; promotes immune function; assists iron absorption.	Exercise increases need for antioxidants; may help reduce free radical damage; protect cell membranes and reduce post-exercise muscle soreness	Fruit and vegetables (e.g. raspberries, blackcurrants, kiwis, oranges, peppers, broccoli, cabbage, tomatoes)	Excess is excreted. Doses over 2 g may lead to diarrhoea and excess urine formation.
Vitamin E	10 mg (EU) SUL = 540 mg	Antioxidant which helps protect against heart disease; promotes normal cell growth and development	Exercise increases need for antioxidants; may help reduce free radical damage, protect cell membranes and reduce post-exercise muscle soreness	Vegetable oils; margarine, oily fish; nuts; seeds; egg yolk; avocado	Toxicity is rare
Calcium	1,000 mg (men) 700 mg (women) SUL = 1,500 mg	Builds bone and teeth; blood clotting; nerve and muscle function	Low oestrogen in female athletes with amenorrhoea increases bone loss and need for calcium	Milk and dairy products; sardines; dark green leafy vegetables; pulses; nuts and seeds	High intakes may interfere with absorption of other minerals. Take with magnesium and vitamin D
Iron	8.7 mg (men) 14.8 mg (women) SUL = 17 mg	Formation of red blood cells; oxygen transport; prevents anaemia	Female athletes may need more to compensate for menstrual losses	Meat and offal; wholegrain cereals; fortified breakfast cereals; pulses; green leafy vegetables	Constipation, stomach discomfort. Avoid unnecessary supplementation – may increase free radical damage
Zinc	9.5 mg (men) 7.0 mg (women) SUL = 25 mg	Healthy immune system; wound healing; skin; cell growth	Exercise increases need for antioxidants; may help immune function	Eggs; wholegrain cereals; meat; milk and dairy products	Interferes with absorption of iron and copper

ESSENTIAL GUIDE TO VITAMINS AND MINERALS (CONTINUED)

Vitamin/mineral	How much? *	Why is it needed?	Benefits	Best food sources	Side effects
Magnesium	300 mg (men) 270 mg (women) SUL = 400 mg	Healthy bones; muscle and nerve function; cell formation	May improve recovery after strength training; increase aerobic capacity	Cereals; fruit; vegetables; milk	Excess may cause diarrhoea
Potassium	3,500 mg SUL = 3,700 mg	Fluid balance; muscle and nerve function	May help prevent cramp	Fruit; vegetables; cereals	Excess is excreted
Selenium	75 µg (men) 60 µg (women) SUL = 350 ug	Antioxidant which helps protect against heart disease and cancer	Exercise increases free radical production	Cereals; vegetables; dairy products; meat; eggs	Excess may cause nausea, vomiting, hair loss

Notes:
mg = milligrams (1,000 mg = 1 gram)
µg = micrograms (1,000 µg = 1 mg)
*The amount needed is given as the Reference Nutrient Intake (RNI, Department of Health, 1991). This is the amount of a nutrient that should cover the needs of 97 per cent of the population. Athletes in hard training may need more.
** SUL = Safe Upper Limit recommended by the Expert Group on Vitamins and Minerals, an independent advisory committee to the Food Standards Agency.

Keep the vitamins in!

■ Buy locally grown produce if you can, ideally from farm shops and local markets.

■ Buy British if you have a choice — imported produce is usually harvested under-ripe (before it has developed its full vitamin quota) and will have lost much of its nutritional value during its journey to your supermarket.

■ Buy unblemished, undamaged fruit and vegetables.

■ Prepare fruit and vegetables just before you make them into a salad or cook them. They start to lose nutrients from the moment they are chopped.

■ Fruit and vegetables should be eaten unpeeled wherever possible – many vitamins and minerals are concentrated just beneath the skin.

■ Use frozen food if fresh is not available as it is nutritionally similar.

■ Cut fruit and vegetables into large pieces rather than small, as vitamins are lost from cut surfaces.

■ Steam or boil vegetables in only the minimum amount of water.

■ When boiling vegetables, add to fast-boiling water and cook as briefly as possible until they are tender-crisp, not soft and mushy.

■ Save the cooking water for soups, stocks and sauces.

■ Do not re-heat leftover cooked vegetables – they will have lost most of their nutritional value.

7. Phytonutrients

What are they?

Phytonutrients are plant compounds that have particular health benefits. They include plant pigments, found in coloured fruit and vegetables, and plant hormones, found in grains, beans, lentils, soya products and herbs.

Many phytonutrients work as antioxidants while others influence enzymes (such as those that block cancer agents). They also:

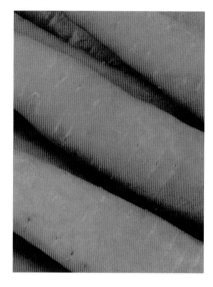

- Fight cancer
- Reduce inflammation
- Combat free radicals
- Lower cholesterol
- Reduce heart disease risk
- Boost immunity
- Balance gut bacteria
- Fight harmful bacteria and viruses

Best sources?

There are hundreds of types of phytonutrients. To make sure you get enough of them eat at least five daily portions of fruits and vegetables, ensuring you include a good range of different colours.

Each colour relates to different phytonutrients in the food, every one having individual health benefits. The more intense the colour, the more phytonutrients you'll be getting. Orange, yellow and red foods (carrots, apricots and mangoes) get their colour from beta-carotene and other carotenoids, while tomatoes and watermelon are rich in lycopene, a type of carotenoid. Carotenoids are powerful antioxidants and help maintain youthful looks. Green foods (broccoli, cabbage, spinach) are rich in magnesium, iron and chlorophyll – a terrific antioxidant. Red/purple foods (plums, cherries, red grapes, blackberries, strawberries) get their colour from anthocyanins, which are even more powerful at fighting harmful free radicals than vitamin C. White foods (apples, pears, cauliflower) contain flavanols, which protect against heart disease and cancer.

WHAT ARE FREE RADICALS?

Free radicals are destructive elements, which are produced continually as a normal part of cell processes. In small numbers they are not a problem. Additional free radicals can be generated by pollution, UV sunlight, cigarette smoke, stress and intense exercise. Left unchecked, they can fur up the arteries and increase the risk of thrombosis, heart disease and cancer. Free radicals are also believed to be partially responsible for post-exercise muscle soreness. The good news is that antioxidants can neutralise them. An antioxidant-rich diet may help protect against these conditions and promote faster recovery after exercise.

8. Antioxidants

What are they?

Antioxidant nutrients include various vitamins such as beta-carotene, vitamin C and vitamin E; minerals such as selenium; and phytonutrients. They are found mostly in fruit and vegetables, seed oils, nuts, whole grains, beans and lentils.

What do they do?

Intense exercise raises levels of harmful free radicals. The body generally produces higher levels of antioxidant enzymes in response to regular exercise, but additional antioxidants from food, or supplements, will help strengthen your defences.

THE ANTIOXIDANT POWER OF FRUIT AND VEGETABLES

Researchers at Tuft's University in Boston, United States, tested various fruits and vegetables for their ability to combat harmful free radicals. They 'scored' each antioxidant with ORAC (Oxygen Radical Absorbance Capacity). All of the foods in the box below left will significantly raise the antioxidant levels in your blood – those at the top will have a greater effect than those at the bottom of the table.

TOP-SCORING ANTIOXIDANT FRUIT AND VEGETABLES

Fruit	ORAC score	Vegetable	ORAC score
Prunes*	5,770	Kale	1,770
Raisins*	2,830	Spinach	1,260
Blueberries	2,400	Brussels sprouts	980
Blackberries	2,036	Alfalfa sprouts	930
Strawberries	1,540	Broccoli	890
Raspberries	1,220	Beets	840
Plums	949	Red peppers	710
Oranges	750	Onions	450
Red grapes	739	Corn	400
Cherries	670	Aubergines	390
Kiwi fruit	602		
Pink grapefruit	483		

Notes:
*The ORAC values of prunes and raisins appear higher because they contain very little water.
Source: Human Nutrition Research Centre on Ageing, Tufts University, Boston, United States.

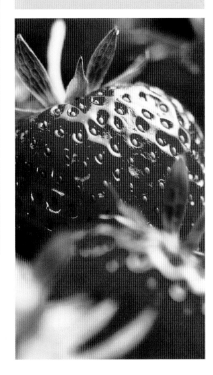

9. Salt

Why do you need it?

Salt is made of sodium and chloride molecules. It is needed for regulating the balance and movement of fluid between cells. Sodium helps cells to absorb nutrients from the blood and also muscles to contract.

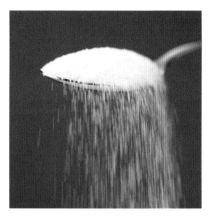

Is too much salt harmful?

While a certain amount of salt is essential, too much can be damaging. Excess sodium can cause raised blood pressure, which triples the risk of heart disease and stroke.

How much?

Try to limit your daily salt intake to 6 g (the UK guideline daily amount) and avoid foods containing more than 1.25 g salt per 100 g.

Seventy-five per cent of the salt we eat comes from processed food, such as meat products (ham, bacon, sausages and burgers), bread, soups, sauces, cheese, ready meals, pizzas, baked beans, breakfast cereals and biscuits. Cutting down on salt reduces blood pressure, whether or not your blood pressure is high to begin with.

Should regular exercisers have extra salt?

Even as a regular exerciser it's unlikely that your salt needs are higher than the average. Salt loss through sweating is relatively small, even when exercising in high temperatures. People in some countries survive on a fraction of the amount of salt eaten by people in the UK. There is no need to consume extra salt – it's more important to drink plenty of water to keep your body hydrated.

10. Water

Why do you need it?

Of all the nutrients, water is the most important. It makes up more than sixty per cent of your body weight and is vital to all cells. Water is the medium in which all metabolic reactions take place, including energy production. Fluid acts as a cushion for your nervous system and acts as a lubricant for your joints and eyes. Blood – another key fluid – carries nutrients and oxygen to the cells and helps rid the body of toxins.

How much?

You need to top up your fluid levels frequently because you lose water through sweat, breathing and urine. Most experts recommend consuming at least 1 litre of water for every 1,000 kcal (4,184 kJ) expended. Since about one-third will come from the food you eat, the British Dietetic Association recommends drinking at least 1.5 litres per day. That's equivalent to roughly six to eight glasses, although you'll need to drink more in hot weather and during exercise. *See* box 'How to keep hydrated', which provides tips on how to drink more water and remain properly hydrated.

11. Alcohol

How much?

The UK Department of Health advises a maximum of 3 units per day and 14 units per week for women; and a maximum of 4 units per day and 21 units per week for men. One unit is equivalent to half a pint of ordinary strength beer or lager, one small glass (125 ml) of wine or one single measure of spirits.

Beneficial or harmful?

Alcohol in moderation is associated with a lowered heart disease risk, due in part to its ability to increase levels of 'good' HDL cholesterol and reduce blood platelet stickiness. Red wine contains polyphenols, saponins and a compound called resveratrol, all of which can help lower 'bad' cholesterol and protect from heart disease.

Do alcohol and exercise mix?

Moderate drinking probably won't jeopardise your exercise performance (provided you don't consume alcohol before training) but you need to account for the calories it provides if you're keeping an eye on your waistline. Two 175 ml glasses of wine will give you 240 calories on top of your daily food calories – the same as a big doughnut. A can of premium lager contains the calorie equivalent of a Danish pastry (260 calories).

Avoid refuelling after exercise with an alcoholic drink. Rehydrate with water or a sports drink before celebrating with lager, beer or shandy, or alternate alcoholic drinks with a glass of water.

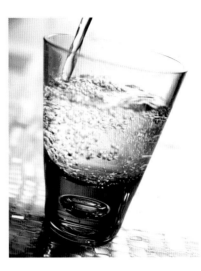

HOW TO KEEP HYDRATED

- Keep a bottle of water on your desk at work.

- Carry a bottle of water with you throughout the day.

- If you don't like the taste of tap water, try bottled water or flavour it with a slice of lemon or lime.

- Drink herbal and fruit teas.

- Have a water break once an hour – set the timer on your watch to remind you to drink.

- Drink water before, during and after working out (*see* chapters 2, 3, and 4 for more information).

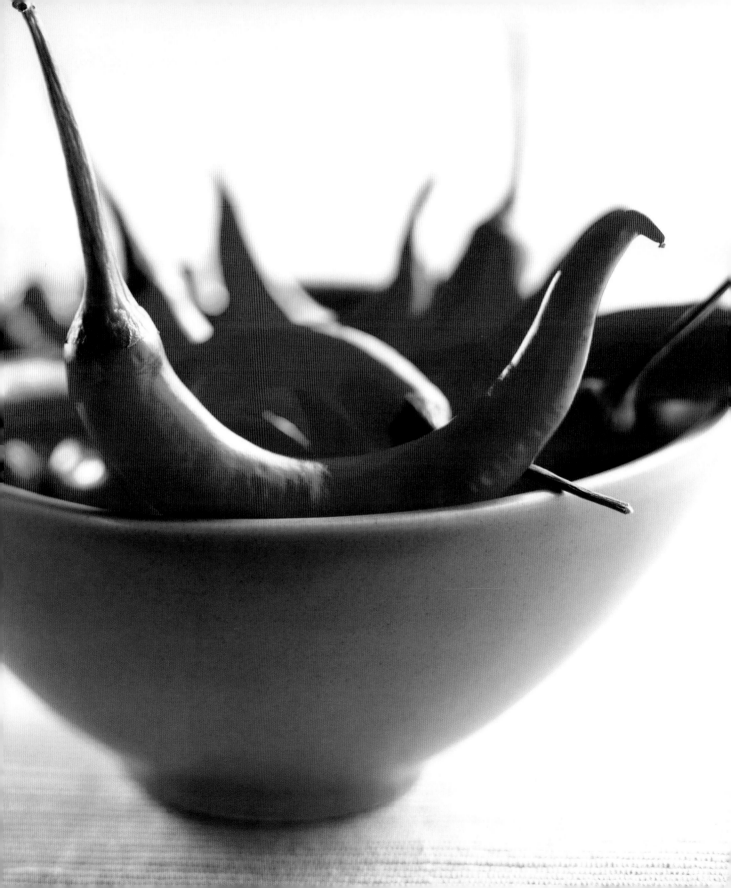

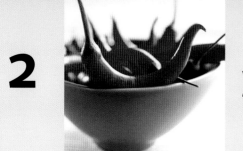

2 your training diet

This chapter provides you with a practical guide to help you put together your daily training diet. I've called it the Fitness Food Pyramid. It is loosely based on the UK's National Food Guide but incorporates up-to-date nutritional advice and provides more realistic portion size guidance suited to the needs of regular exercisers. In line with the new US dietary guidelines and the latest research from Harvard University, the Pyramid recommends eating more fruit and vegetables, whole grains and healthy fats. It also discourages saturated fats, trans fats and refined carbohydrates such as white bread. The chances are that UK authorities will eventually incorporate many of these recommendations into their own guidelines.

How to use the Fitness Food Pyramid

Use the Fitness Food Pyramid to devise your daily menu or to check your current eating plan.

The foods in the lower layers of the pyramid should form the main part of your diet while those at the top should be eaten in smaller quantities.

■ Include foods from each group in the pyramid each day.

■ Make sure you include a variety of foods within each group.

■ Aim to include the suggested number of portions from each food group each day.

■ Check the portion sizes suggested in the 'What Counts as a Portion?' box, page 29.

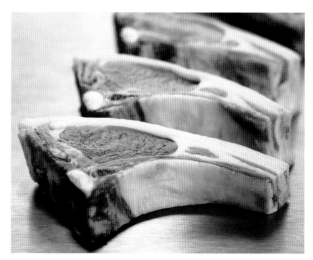

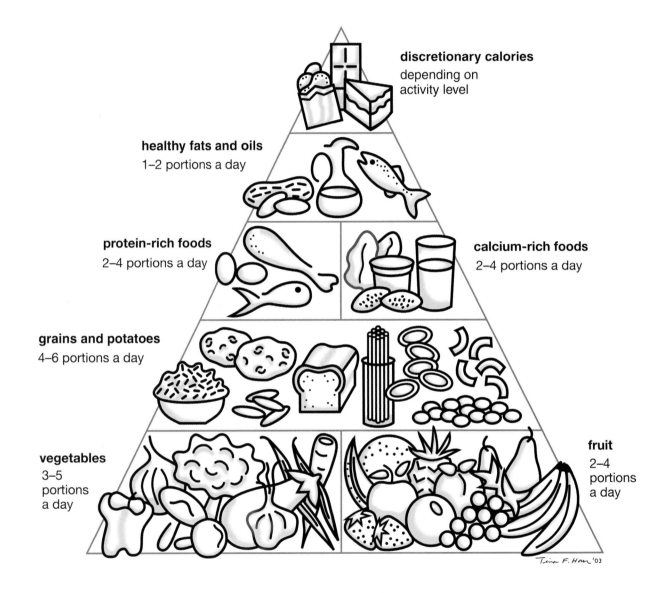

food *for* fitness

discretionary calories
depending on
activity level

healthy fats and oils
1–2 portions a day

protein-rich foods
2–4 portions a day

calcium-rich foods
2–4 portions a day

grains and potatoes
4–6 portions a day

vegetables
3–5
portions
a day

fruit
2–4
portions
a day

28

WHAT COUNTS AS A PORTION?

Food Group	Number of portions each day	Food	Portion size
Vegetables	*3–5*	***1 portion = 80 g (amount you can hold in the palm of your hand)***	
		Broccoli, cauliflower	2–3 spears/florets
		Carrots	1 carrot
		Other vegetables and salad	2 tablespoons
		Tomatoes	5 cherry tomatoes
Fruit	*2–4*	***1 portion = 80 g (size of a tennis ball)***	
		Apple, pear, peach, banana	1 medium fruit
		Plum, kiwi fruit, satsuma	1–2 fruit
		Strawberries	8–10
		Grapes	12–16
		Tinned fruit	3 tablespoons
		Fruit juice	1 medium glass
Grains and potatoes 4–6		***1 portion = (size of your clenched fist)***	
		Bread	2 slices (60 g)
		Roll/bagel/wrap	1 item (60 g)
		Pasta or rice	5 tablespoons (180 g)
		Breakfast cereal	1 bowl (40–50 g)
		Potatoes, sweet potatoes, yams	1 fist-sized (150 g)
Calcium-rich foods	*2–4*	***1 portion = 200 ml milk***	
		Milk (dairy or calcium-fortified soya milk)	1 medium cup (200 ml)
		Cheese	Size of 4 dice (40 g)
		Tofu	Size of 4 dice (60 g)
		Yoghurt/fromage frais	1 pot (150 ml)
Protein-rich foods	*2–4*	***1 portion = size of a deck of cards (70 g)***	
		Lean meat	3 slices
		Poultry	2 medium slices/1 breast
		Fish	1 fillet (115–140 g)
		Egg	2
		Lentils/beans	5 tablespoons (150 g)
		Tofu/soya burger or sausage	1–2
Healthy fats and oils	*1–2*	***1 portion = 1 tablespoon***	
		Nuts and seeds	2 tablespoons (25 g)
		Seed oils, nut oils	1 tablespoon (15 ml)
		Avocado	Half avocado
		Oily fish*	Deck of cards (140 g)
Discretionary calories	*Depending on calorie expenditure*	*Sugars and sugary foods: jam, desserts, cakes, biscuits, sweets, chocolates, soft drinks, sports drinks, energy bars, Alcoholic drinks*	*Depending on calorie expenditure*

*Oily fish is very rich in essential fats so just 1 portion a week would cover your needs

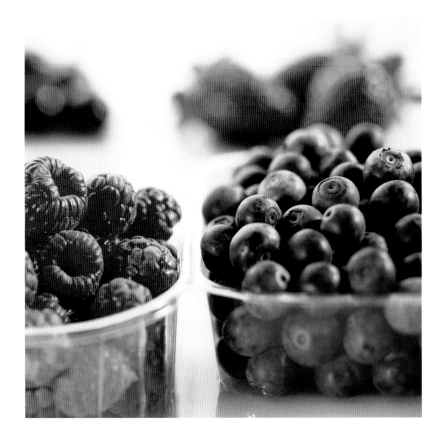

Fruit and vegetables

3–5 portions of vegetables a day
2–4 portions of fruit a day

Research indicates that people who have a high level of fruit and vegetables in their diet have lower risks of cancer, heart disease, stroke and bowel disease. That's because fruit and vegetables are packed with vitamins, minerals, fibre and phytonutrients, which are vital for peak health. For regular exercisers, eating more fruit and veg means you'll take in more vitamins such as vitamin C to help aid recovery from tough workouts and minerals such as potassium and magnesium for healthy fluid balance and bones.

Grains and potatoes

4–6 daily portions

This group includes foods rich in complex carbohydrates: breads, breakfast cereal, rice, pasta, porridge oats, beans, lentils and potatoes. These foods are also major sources of fibre, B vitamins (such as thiamin and niacin) and minerals (such as iron). Focus on wholegrain varieties, such as wholemeal bread, breakfast cereals, pasta and rice, rather than refined 'white' versions, which have been largely stripped of vitamins, minerals and fibre. Studies show that people who consume more wholegrains are 49 per cent less likely to be overweight than those who consume the least and have a lower risk of heart disease, diabetes and certain cancers. There are no formal recommendations for wholegrains in the UK but the US government recommends three 16 g servings a day.

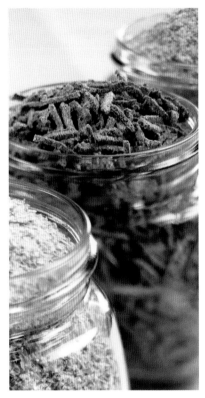

MAKE IT HAPPEN!

- Opt for breakfast cereals labelled wholegrain, for example bran flakes, Shreddies, muesli, Shredded Wheat or Weetabix.

- Swap white bread for wholegrain breads (such as wholemeal, rye, oatmeal), wholegrain crackers and biscuits.

- Use whole grains in one-pot dishes such as barley in vegetable soup or stews and bulgur wheat in casseroles or stir-fries. Create a whole grain pilaf with a mixture of barley, wild rice, brown rice, stock and herbs. Then add toasted nuts or chopped dried fruit.

- Add wholemeal flour or oatmeal when making cakes, muffins or fruit crumbles.

Calcium-rich foods

2–4 portions a day

Including dairy products (milk, cheese, yoghurt, and fromage frais) in your daily diet is the easiest way to get your calcium, which is needed for strong bones and teeth, heart health and, according to a study at Colorado University, can also help burn body fat. As a bonus, you'll also be getting protein and B vitamins. If you don't like dairy foods, make sure you choose alternative calcium sources, such as almonds, dark green vegetables, tinned fish with soft bones (such as sardines, salmon), calcium-fortified juices, soya milk, tofu, pulses and figs.

MAKE IT HAPPEN!

- Start your day with one serving of dairy or the equivalent. A breakfast of cereal and milk, porridge made with milk, yogurt and fruit, or a smoothie made with yoghurt or soya milk gives you a good part of your daily allotment.

- Use yoghurt as a base for salad dressings. Flavour with fresh herbs, such as mint or coriander, lemon or lime juice, and use for dipping fresh vegetables.

- Top casseroles, soups, stews, or vegetables with grated cheese. Top baked potatoes with yoghurt or fromage frais.

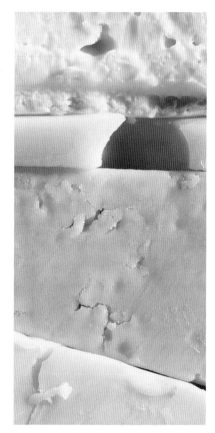

Protein-rich foods

2–4 portions a day

This group includes meat, poultry, fish, eggs, beans, lentils, soya, and quorn. Protein-rich foods are not only rich in protein but are also good sources of B vitamins, iron and zinc. Vegetarians may also count dairy foods toward their protein target. Protein supplements can also be included in this group if you struggle to get enough protein from your food. Regular exercisers need more protein than inactive people. Without enough protein, you'll take longer to recover after training and your strength and muscle gains will be slower.

MAKE IT HAPPEN!

- Ensure at least half of your protein quota comes from plant sources such as beans, lentils and soya. They supply fibre and various phytonutrients beneficial for heart health and cancer prevention.

- Keep your saturated fat intake in check by opting for leaner cuts of meat, trimming off any visible fat, removing the skin from chicken or turkey and rejecting fatty processed meats such as burgers, sausages and coated or fried products.

- Include beans and lentils in soups, salads, curries and pilaffs. Add to Bolognese sauce, stews, chilli and shepherd's pie.

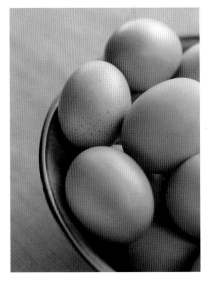

Healthy fats
1–2 portions a day

Most of your fat intake should come from monounsaturated and polyunsaturated sources. This group includes nuts, seeds, all seed and nut oils (e.g. rapeseed, olive, walnut, flaxseed, sesame, sunflower oils), avocado, and oily fish (including salmon, sardines, trout, herring, fresh (not tinned) tuna, and mackerel). These foods contain high levels of 'good' fats, the omega-3 and omega-6 fatty acids, which protect against heart disease and stroke. For regular exercisers, eating more omega-3 fats can help improve endurance, aid recovery and boost the immune system.

MAKE IT HAPPEN!

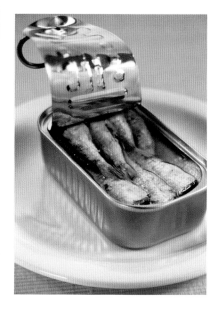

- Include at least one portion (140 g) a week of oily fish such as mackerel or salmon. The FSA advise women who are pregnant or breast-feeding not to eat more than two portions a week (fish may contain dioxins and PCBs) but those not planning to become pregnant may eat up to four weekly portions.

- Add nuts, pumpkin seeds and flax seeds (linseeds) to breakfast cereals, muesli, yoghurt, shakes and smoothies. You'll need to grind flaxseeds in a coffee grinder to benefit from the oils as the tough outer husk is practically impenetrable by digestive enzymes.

- Use omega-3-rich cold-pressed oils in dressings. Don't fry with these oils, as high temperatures will reduce their nutritional value. Blend into soups, casseroles and sauces after cooking.

Discretionary calories

Discretionary calories are what you have left after you have met your daily targets for fruit and vegetables, grains, protein-rich and calcium-rich foods and healthy fats. The more active you are, the more discretionary calories are allowed. For most regular exercisers this is likely to be around 200–300 calories worth of treats such as biscuits, cakes, puddings, alcoholic drinks, chocolate or crisps. But these extra calories also need to account for any added sugar in sports drinks and energy bars consumed.

The UK Food Standards Agency advises eating no more than 10 per cent of total calories from added sugars, that's equivalent to 65 g daily for a person on a 2,500 kcal diet.

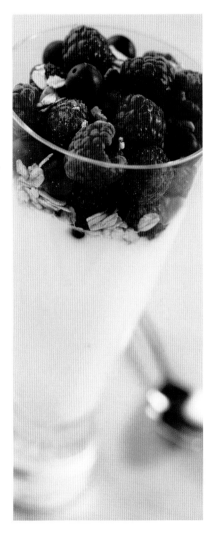

MAKE IT HAPPEN!

■ Limit your sugars to only your favourite treats, then select one each day. Omit the sugar in your breakfast cereal in favour of your after-dinner scoop of ice cream.

■ Fruit can satisfy a sweet tooth. Snack on grapes, apples, pineapple or mango when you feel the need for something sweet.

■ If you must have something sugary, pick foods that are also loaded with other nutrients, such as low-fat fruit yogurt, chocolate-covered nuts, low-fat frozen yogurt, ice cream, fruit cake, malt loaf, a cereal bar (without hydrogenated oils), dark chocolate containing 70 per cent cocoa solids, fig rolls, milkshake or rice pudding.

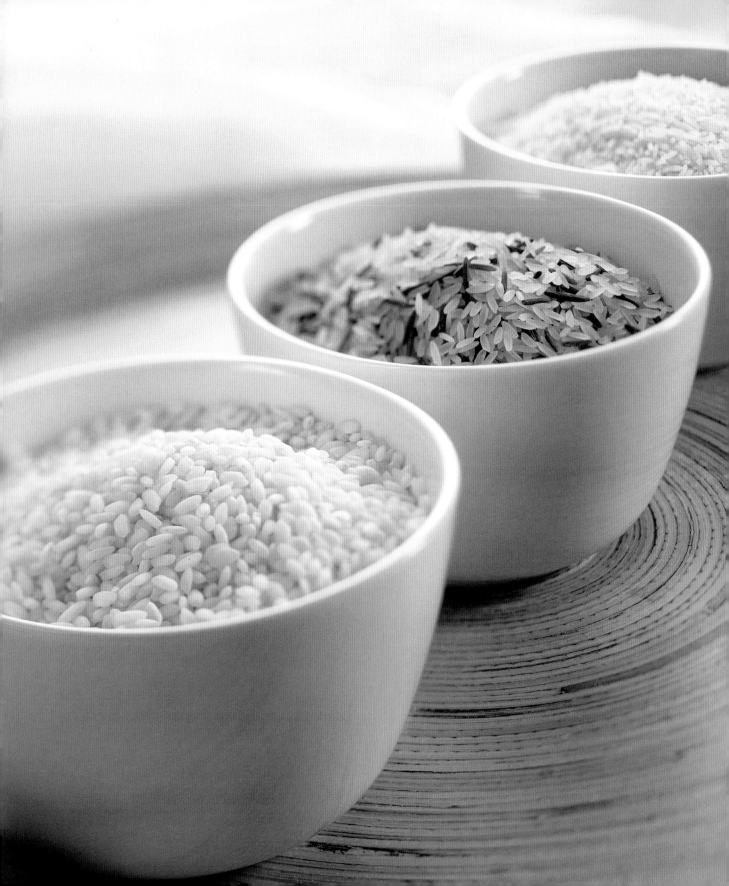

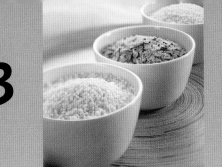

3　before training

What you eat and drink the day before and during the several hours before your workout dictates how much energy you'll have for training and how well you will perform. It also affects how much body fat, glycogen or even muscle tissue you burn. Get it wrong and you may find yourself struggling to complete your planned workout and performing under-par. Even worse, you could end up burning muscle rather than fat as your fuel reserves dip.

Get your pre-exercise nutrition right and you'll have plenty of energy to train hard and perform at your best. Eating the right amount and type of carbohydrate as well as timing your pre-exercise meal correctly will help avoid common problems such as fatigue, dizziness, fainting and stitch. This chapter guides you through a practical pre-exercise eating and drinking strategy.

Why eat before training?

The main purpose of your pre-workout meal is to stabilise your blood sugar levels during exercise. It also staves off hunger and minimises the risk of problems such as stitch and hypoglycaemia (low blood sugar levels).

But don't expect your pre-workout meal to fuel your muscles. There isn't enough time for your body to turn the food into glycogen – the muscles' main fuel supply – so your body must rely on existing glycogen (and fat) stores.

It takes 24 hours to refill muscle glycogen stores, so what you've consumed the previous day matters. For most regular exercisers, a daily diet providing carbohydrates of around 280–350 g for a 70 kg person (*see* 'How much carbohydrate?' page 4) will satisfy muscle glycogen levels.

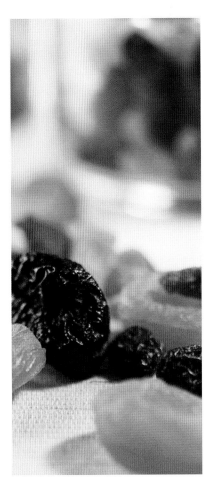

Should you train on empty?

It is definitely not advisable to train on an empty stomach, especially if you want to improve strength, endurance or performance.

Firstly, you're more likely to feel lethargic and unmotivated when you haven't eaten for several hours. Eating a light snack a couple of hours before your workout will reduce the temptation to skip your training.

Secondly, when your brain isn't getting enough fuel you'll feel faint, lose concentration and risk injury. You may become light-headed, weak and shaky – all symptoms of low blood sugar levels – and this will certainly stop you from working out.

Finally, you are more likely to fatigue early as muscle glycogen and blood sugar levels dip. Rather like a car running out of petrol, your body will come to a weary halt. You wouldn't take your car out on a long journey when the petrol tank is low. So you can't expect to exercise very hard or very long when you haven't fuelled your body for several hours.

How much to eat before training

The exact amount you should eat depends on your body weight (heavier people need more) and how hard and long you plan to exercise (eat more for longer, harder workouts). In general, if you plan to workout for less than 2 hours, aim to eat around 1 g carbohydrate per kg of body weight (or 70 g for a 70 kg person) or 400–600 calories. For longer workouts or endurance events eat around 2 g carbohydrate per kg of body weight (or 600–800 calories).

Don't eat a big meal just before a workout otherwise you will feel uncomfortable, sluggish and 'heavy'.

When to eat before training

Ideally, you should aim to have a meal 2–4 hours before a workout. This should leave enough time to partially digest your food although, in practice, the exact timing of your pre-workout meal may depend on your daily schedule. You should feel comfortable – neither full nor hungry.

According to a study at the University of North Carolina, United States, eating a moderately-high carbohydrate, low fat meal 3 hours before exercise allows you to exercise longer and perform better.

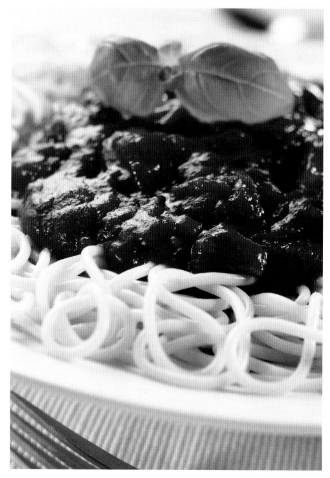

Researchers asked a group of athletes to eat a meal both 3 hours and 6 hours before the experiments. The athletes were then asked to run on treadmills for periods of 30 minutes without breaks; first at moderate intensity, then switching to high intensity, until they couldn't run any further. The athletes ran for much longer periods after eating the meal 3 hours before training compared with when they had eaten 6 hours before.

Q&A

Question: *I like to run first thing in the morning. Should I force myself to eat?*

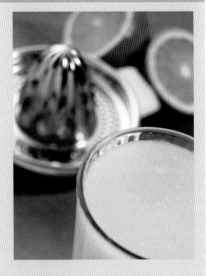

Answer: Many runners claim they can't run with food in their stomachs, complaining of stitch, nausea or stomach discomfort. It is down to individual preference, but it is possible to 'train' yourself to run with a small amount of food inside you. The potential benefits are more energy and greater endurance.

Try different high carb options to find what works for you, such as a slice of toast, a banana, a small cereal or energy bar, a pot of yoghurt or a handful of dried fruit (such as raisins, apricots or sultanas). If you can't face solid food, try a liquid meal: fruit juice (diluted half and half with water), a smoothie, flavoured milk or a commercial carbohydrate and protein shake. Ensure you drink a cupful (150–250 ml) of water or diluted juice before setting out. This will help rehydrate you after your night's fast and reduce the risk of dehydration during your workout. If you cannot eat anything at all, make sure that you eat plenty the day before and for breakfast after your workout.

DOES EXERCISING ON AN EMPTY STOMACH HELP BURN MORE FAT?

Many people believe that training on empty will help them shed weight faster. It is actually better to eat a light snack 2–4 hours before exercise. The resulting rise in blood glucose levels slows the rate of glycogen depletion, enabling you to exercise harder and longer, and to therefore burn more calories.

According to University of Connecticut researchers, the downside of exercising on an empty stomach is that you fatigue sooner and/or exercise at a lower intensity, so you end up burning fewer calories than if you had grabbed a snack before working out. Exercising in a fasted state may reduce your endurance and encourage your muscles to turn to protein for fuel, so you can literally burn away muscle fibres!

What are the best foods to eat just before a workout?

Slow-burning or low-GI foods – that is, foods that produce a gradual rise in blood sugar levels (*see* pages 4–7) – are the best foods before a workout. Studies at the University of Sydney, Australia, have found that athletes who ate a low-GI meal before exercise were able to keep going considerably longer than those who ate a high-GI meal. It seems that low-GI foods help spare muscle glycogen and avoid problems of low blood sugar levels during long training sessions.

Low-GI meals may also help you burn more fat during exercise. A 2003 study at Loughborough University, UK, found that runners who ate a low-GI meal 3 hours before exercise burned more fat than those who ate a high-GI meal with the same amount of carbs.

Remember, a low-GI meal can either be low-GI carbs, such as fruit and yoghurt or higher-GI foods combined with protein and/or fat, such as Weetabix with milk or a baked potato with cheese (*see* page 41 'Pre-exercise snacks and meals' for more suggestions).

Alternatively, modest portions of high-GI foods, such as confectionery, can be eaten before exercise. While these foods have a high GI, if you eat them in small amounts, you'll get only a low or moderate glycaemic load (GL) ie. a small or moderate rise in blood sugar (*see* box below 'Will eating a few sweets before training give me a quick energy fix?').

Q&A

Question: *Will eating a few sweets before training give me a quick energy fix?*

Answer: Sweets have a high GI and can raise blood sugar levels rapidly. Providing you have only a small amount, this could be beneficial for exercise. For example, a small portion of jellybeans (25 g sugar per 30 g portion) will produce only a moderate blood sugar rise or GL (*see* pages 7–8) of 19, despite its high GI (76). Double your portion size to 60 g (or 50 g sugar) and you'll get a GL of 38 – enough to send your blood sugar levels soaring.

This carries a big risk of hypoglycaemia (low blood sugar), faintness and dizziness, especially if it strikes while you're exercising. Therefore, stick to small portions of high GL sugary foods (such as sweets, chocolate and even dried fruit) before working out or opt for lower GL choices such as bananas, grapes or yoghurt drinks.

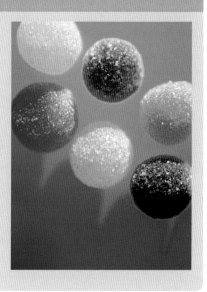

Pre-exercise meals

The following meals have a low or moderate GI and produce a low or moderate GL. Eat 2–4 hours before exercise:

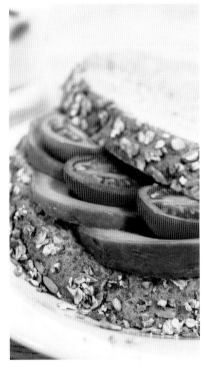

- Sandwich/roll/bagel/wrap filled with chicken, fish, cheese, egg or peanut butter
- Jacket potato with beans, cheese, tuna, coleslaw or chicken
- Pasta with tomato-based pasta sauce, vegetables and cheese
- Macaroni cheese with salad
- Rice with chicken or fish and vegetables
- Porridge made with milk
- Wholegrain cereal (e.g. bran or wheat flakes, muesli or Weetabix) with milk or yoghurt
- Fish pie (fish in sauce with mashed potatoes)
- Noodles with stir-fried prawns (or tofu) and vegetables.

Pre-workout snacks

The following snacks have a low or moderate GI and produce a low or moderate GL. Eat up to 1 hour before exercise:

- 2–3 portions (200–300 g) fresh fruit, e.g. grapes, apples, peaches, apricots
- 1–2 bananas
- Approximately 40 g raisins, dried apricots or sultanas
- One 300 ml smoothie (homemade or ready-bought)
- 1 or 2 pots (150–300 ml) fruit yoghurt
- 1 large glass (250 ml) flavoured milk or shake (homemade or ready-bought)
- 1 small (50 g) energy or sports bar
- 1 (30 g) cereal bar or breakfast bar
- 1 large glass (250 ml) fruit juice
- 3 rice cakes, thinly spread with peanut butter

Q&A

Question: *What should I eat before a competition?*

Answer: You should take your own supplies for the journey as well for race day as suitable foods may not be available. Keep to the guidelines for training outlined above, but keep in mind that competition nerves may reduce your appetite or affect your digestion (*see* chapter xx for more pre-event advice). In general:

■ Stick to familiar foods – don't try anything new.

■ Be certain that what you're eating and drinking is uncontaminated and safe.

■ Drink plenty of water.

■ Avoid high-fat, salty or very sugary foods.

■ Eat little and often (*see* suggestions for pre-workout snacks, page 41).

■ Liquid meals such as shakes, smoothies and juices may be more palatable than solid food.

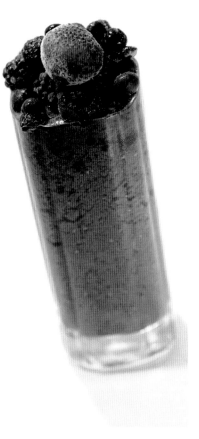

Why drink before training?

It is important to ensure that you are properly hydrated before training to minimise the risk of dehydration during exercise. Even mild dehydration can result in early fatigue as your body is unable to cool itself efficiently, which puts extra stress on the heart and lungs. Exercise feels tougher when you are dehydrated and you cannot train as hard. The dangers of dehydration during exercise are explained in chapter 4 (*see* pages 47–52).

When to drink before training?

The best strategy is to keep hydrated throughout the day rather than load up with fluid just before your workout. Try to make a habit of drinking water regularly. Have a glass of water first thing in the morning and then schedule drinks during your day. Aim for at least 8 glasses (1½–2) daily, and more in hot weather or workout days.

It's better to drink little and often rather than drinking large amounts in one go, which promotes urination and a greater loss of fluid. Carry a bottle of water with you everywhere: to the gym, office and in the car, as a constant reminder to drink. It need not be expensive bottled water. A simple water bottle or a bottled-water bottle will do – just refill with tap water.

Drink before you get thirsty. By the time your thirst mechanism kicks in you may have lost around 2 per cent of your body weight as water. If you relied on your thirst alone, you would replace only 50–75 per cent of the amount you need.

How much to drink before training?

The American College of Sports Medicine Drink recommends drinking 2–4 glasses of water (400–600 ml) during the 2–3 hours before you workout. Don't drink it all in one go – divide into several smaller amounts and sip at regular intervals.

Q&A

Question: *How can I tell if I'm dehydrated?*

Answer: Checking your urine is the easiest way to assess your body's hydration. Dark gold-coloured urine is a sure sign that you're low on fluid. Drink plenty of water and aim for light yellow-coloured urine. You should pass urine at least 8 times daily when you are well hydrated.

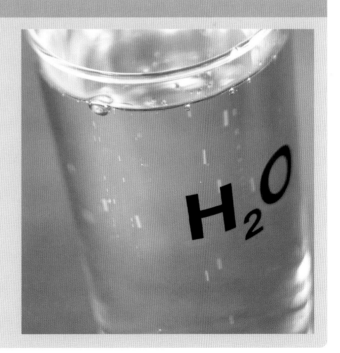

Q&A

Question: *Do coffee and tea dehydrate rather than rehydrate you?*

Answer: Coffee and tea contain caffeine, which is a mild diuretic, but they do not dehydrate the body, as was once thought. According to several US studies drinking caffeine-containing drinks immediately before a workout won't cause dehydration nor have any detrimental effect on your performance (indeed, it may even enhance your endurance). But, at rest, caffeine drinks may 'make you go' more frequently.

A daily intake of 3 cups of coffee (less than 300 mg of caffeine) results in no larger urine output than water, according to University of Connecticut researchers. At this level, caffeine is considered safe and unlikely to affect your performance or health.

Drinking coffee and tea regularly builds up your caffeine tolerance, so you experience smaller diuretic effects.

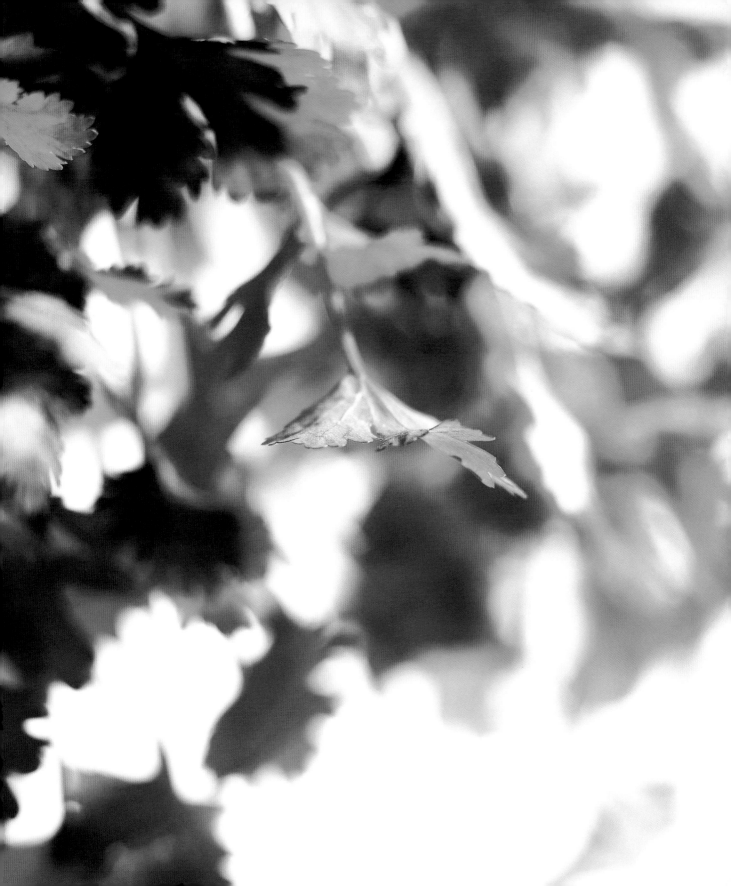

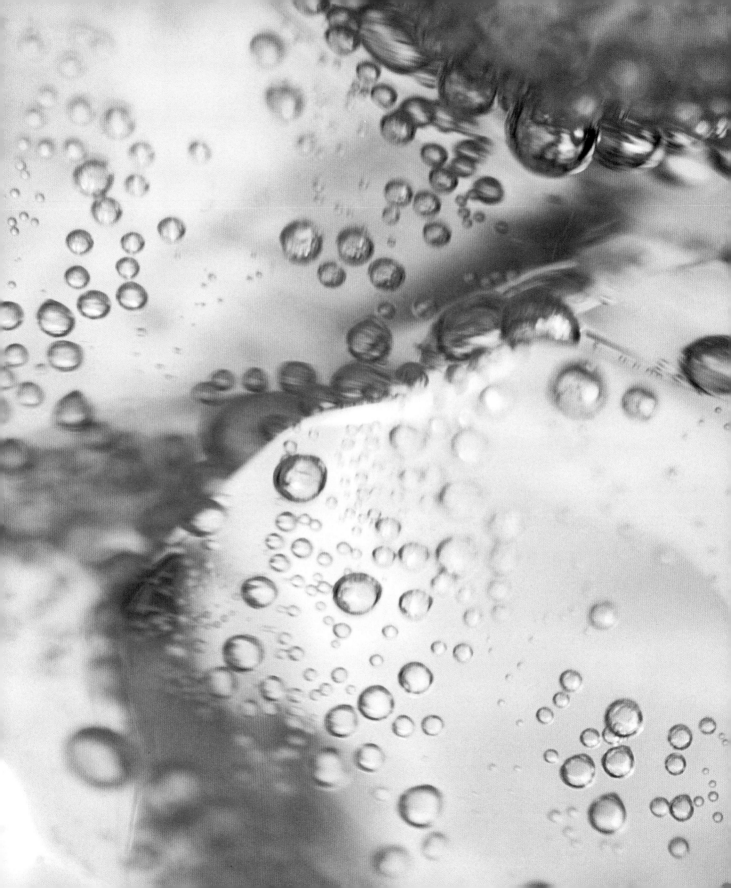

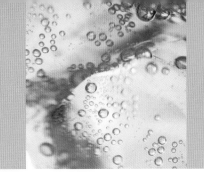

4   during training

Everyone exercising for longer than 30 minutes will certainly benefit from drinking something during exercise. But with the growing array of sports drinks, sports 'waters' and energy drinks it's a confusing choice for most regular exercisers.

If you plan to exercise longer than 60 minutes, you may also benefit from additional carbohydrate. But should you take carbohydrates in liquid or solid form? Exactly how much and when? This chapter provides the answers to help you fuel on the move.

Why sweat during training?

As soon as you begin exercising, you lose fluid in the form of sweat. Sweating is a vital function. It rids your body of excess heat produced during exercise, maintaining your core body temperature. Without sweating you would quickly over-heat and die.

But fluid losses can be high – up to 500 ml in 30 minutes – depending on how hard and long you are training as well as the surrounding temperature and humidity. Also, heavier people sweat more and some people simply sweat more than others.

Why drink during training?

If you don't replace at least some of your sweat losses, your core temperature will rise and your cardiovascular system will have to work much harder than normal. Your blood will become more viscous (or 'thicker') and your heart will need to beat faster to pump the blood around your body.

Losing the equivalent of 2 per cent of your body weight in sweat results in a 10–20 per cent drop in your performance (or aerobic capacity). When you become dehydrated, exercise feels harder, endurance is reduced and you will fatigue sooner. In severe cases, it can result in vomiting and heat exhaustion.

It is a myth that you can 'train' yourself to exercise without drinking much or that you can adapt to dehydration. You increase the risk of health problems and should not ignore the warning signs (*see* box 'Warning signs of dehydration on page 48).

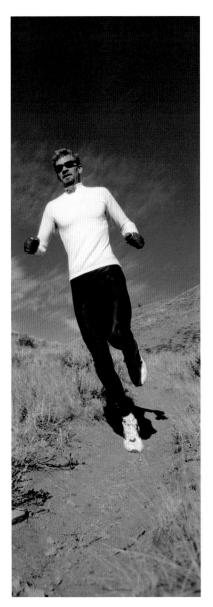

WARNING SIGNS OF DEHYDRATION

Early symptoms:

- Unusually lacking in energy
- Fatiguing early during exercise
- Feeling too hot
- Skin appears flushed and feels cool and clammy
- Passing only small volumes of dark-coloured urine
- Nausea

Action: Stop exercising. Drink 100–200 ml water or sports drink every 10–15 minutes.

Advanced symptoms:

- A bad headache
- Becoming dizzy or light-headed
- Appearing disorientated
- Short of breath

Action: Stop exercising. Drink 100–200 ml of sports drink every 10–15 minutes. Seek professional help.

THE AFFECTS OF DEHYDRATION

- Increases core body temperature
- Exercise feels much harder
- Increases heart rate
- Can cause cramp, headaches and nausea
- Reduces concentration
- Decreases your ability to perform sports skills
- Makes you fatigue sooner and lose stamina

Water those muscles

Dehydration not only reduces your endurance, but also saps your strength. Researchers at the Old Dominion University in Virginia, United States, tested the strength of ten young weight trainers on the bench press following dehydration. The amount of weight they could lift was significantly lower (by about 6 kg) when they were dehydrated compared to when they were rehydrated. So water those muscles and watch them grow!

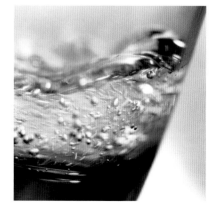

How much to drink?

During exercise you should aim to match your fluid intake as closely as possible to your loss. Studies with athletes at the University of Aberdeen, Scotland, have shown that if you can replace at least 80 per cent of your fluid loss or keep within 1 per cent of your body weight (*see* box 'Working out how much to drink', below), then your performance won't suffer.

Exactly how much you need to drink depends on how heavily you are sweating. If you're exercising hard in warm conditions, you can count on losing around 750–1,000 ml per hour so you'll need to put back around 600–800 ml in that time. You'll need to schedule in drink breaks and learn to drink on the run. If you can only manage a few sips at a time, then make sure they are frequent. The American College of Sports Medicine and American Dietetics Association recommend drinking 150–350 ml every 15–20 minutes. In practice, aim to take about six big gulps every 15–20 minutes (*see* chapter 9 for practical tips on drinking and eating on the move while running, cycling and swimming).

You should start drinking early during your workout as it takes about 30 minutes for the fluid to be absorbed into your bloodstream. **Don't wait until you feel thirsty as this indicates that you are already on your way to dehydration!**

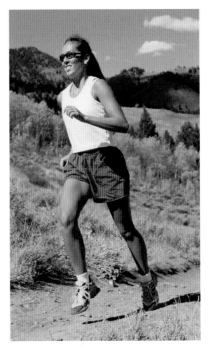

Working out how much to drink

To work out how much fluid you lose in a typical workout and, therefore, how much you ought to drink, weigh yourself before and after exercising. You can assume that all of your weight loss is fluid. A weight loss of 0.5 kg represents a fluid loss of 500 ml. Aim to replace that fluid loss with one and a half times that volume of fluid. This accounts for the fact that you continue sweating after exercise and that urination usually increases during this time. So, if you have lost 0.5 kg, you should aim to drink 750 ml of fluid during and after your workout. Divide this volume into manageable amounts, according to the activity you are doing. For example, you may drink 125 ml (about half a cup) four times during your workout, and a further 250 ml (1 cup) immediately after your workout.

What to drink?

Workouts lasting less than 1 hour

For most activities, water is all you need. It is absorbed relatively quickly into your bloodstream and keeps your body hydrated. It's cheap, plentiful and readily available.

If you're not keen on the taste of water and cannot force enough down, flavour it with a little cordial, fruit juice or high-juice squash. This will introduce extra sugar (carbohydrate) but provided it's well diluted it won't harm your performance. Sugar-free drinks don't contain any carbohydrates but include artificial sweeteners and other artificial additives, which you may prefer to avoid. Sports or fitness 'waters' provide low levels of sugar (around 2 g per 100 ml) as well as sodium to help replace sweat losses, but are also packed with artificial additives.

Workouts lasting more than 1 hour

Drinks containing carbohydrates – isotonic sports drinks, diluted juice and high-juice squash – are better than plain water when you are working out hard for longer than 60 minutes. The sugars they contain not only provide fuel for your exercising muscles but also speed up the absorption of water into your bloodstream. Ideally, you should aim to consume 30–60 g of carbohydrate per hour, depending on how hard you are exercising. That's equivalent to 500 ml–1 l of an isotonic sports drink or fruit juice diluted 50/50 with water (both equivalent to 6 g sugar per 100 ml.)

Why choose sports drinks?

The main benefits of sports drinks are their sugar content, which speeds the absorption of water, tops up blood sugar levels and provides extra fuel for long hard workouts, and their sodium content, which increases the urge to drink and improves the drink's taste.

Commercial brands are essentially mixtures of sugars (glucose, sucrose, fructose, maltodextrins or a combination of these) and mineral salts, or electrolytes (sodium, potassium, magnesium and chloride). They may also provide certain vitamins, artificial sweeteners, colours and preservatives. The additives in sports drinks – as with any food or drink – are considered safe but you may wish to avoid high levels, as the long-term risks (particularly of

Q&A

Question: *Which are better for rehydrating you: cold or warm drinks?*

Answer: It was thought that cold drinks were better at hydrating you than ambient or warm ones. However, a study from the University of Minas Gerais, Brazil, challenges this idea. Cyclists took the same time to reach fatigue whether they drank cold, warm or hot water. What is important is how much you drink. Colder drinks are generally more palatable, helping you to drink more.

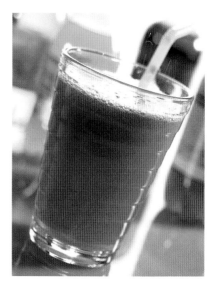

additive combinations) are unknown. Other mineral salts and vitamins have no immediate effect on your performance and simply add to your overall daily intake.

The sugar concentration may be either **_isotonic_** (the same concentration as body fluids) or **_hypotonic_** (more dilute than body fluids, usually branded as 'fitness water' or 'light'). Both are absorbed into the bloodstream slightly faster than plain water. Which type you opt for depends on how hard and long you're exercising and therefore how much extra carbohydrate you need.

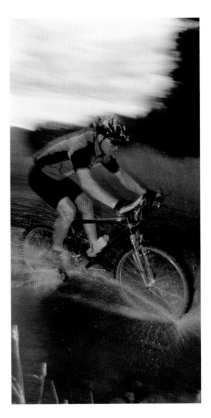

WHAT'S IN SPORT'S DRINKS?

Glucose – the basic sugar unit and the body's immediate source of cellular energy

Sucrose – ordinary white sugar, consisting of glucose and fructose together

Fructose – fruit sugar that tastes sweeter than sucrose and produces a smaller blood sugar rise

Maltodextrin (glucose polymer) – produced commercially from cornstarch; comprises between 4 and 20 glucose units. Is much less sweet than sucrose.

Aspartame – low-cal sweetener up to 200 times sweeter than sugar. High intakes have been linked with headaches, migraines and depression, and a 2006 European study linked Aspartame to cancer in lab rats.

Do sports drinks work?

Sports drinks, commercial or home-made, may help improve your endurance during activities lasting longer than 60 minutes. Research from the University of Texas, United States, found that drinking water during 1 hour of cycling improved performance by 6 per cent compared with no water, but drinking a sport's drink resulted in a 12 per cent improvement on performance. Researchers at the University of Loughborough, England, found that when runners drank a sports drink (containing 5.5 g carbohydrate per 100 ml), they improved their running time by 3.9 minutes over 42 km compared with drinking water.

MAKE YOUR OWN SPORTS DRINK

■ 500 ml fruit juice mixed with 500 ml water and one-eighth of a teaspoon salt (optional).

■ 200 ml squash (preferably organic or without artificial sweeteners and additives) mixed with 800 ml water and 0.5–0.7 g (one eighth of a teaspoon) salt (optional).

Is it possible to drink too much water?

It is possible, though not common, to over-hydrate. Drinking too much water causes 'hyponatraemia', or water intoxication. This can happen during events lasting several hours – such as cycling, marathon running and hiking – when you lose a lot of sweat and drink water all the time. Excessive sweating combined with drinking only water dilutes the concentration of salts in the body to a dangerously low level. The result is nausea, lethargy, dizziness and mental confusion: it's possible to lapse into a coma. If you plan to exercise for more than 4 hours in warm weather, drink no more than 800 ml per hour, be guided by thirst (instead of forcing yourself to drink) and sip a sports drink containing sugar and salt.

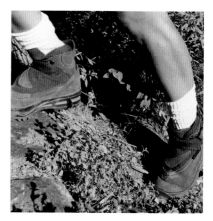

Q&A

Question: *Many athletes swear by fizzy cola during races. Does it really improve your performance?*

Answer: Cola is a very popular drink among athletes, but this is often due to the taste rather than the carbonation. Drinking cola is not necessarily a bad thing since athletes tend to drink more of anything they find palatable. It is also possible that the caffeine in cola enhances performance, by increasing fatty acid levels in the blood and increasing endurance.

Researchers at Washington University School of Medicine, United States, addressed the question of carbonation. In their study, cyclists were given fizzy or flat drinks containing either 10 per cent carbohydrates or no carbohydrates on four separate occasions. The investigators found that both the fizzy and flat drinks emptied from the stomach at the same speed, and in the case of the 10 per cent carb drinks raised blood sugar levels to a similar extent. In other words, carbonation has no detrimental or beneficial effect on a drink's ability to rehydrate the body during exercise or deliver carbs to exercising muscles.

Another team of US researchers looked at the effect of fizzy versus flat sports drinks on runners. Again, rehydration was equal, but runners were more likely to complain of mild heartburn and stomach discomfort when drinking fizzy drinks containing 8 g carbohydrate per 100 ml as opposed to calorie-free ones. Despite this, the amount of fluid consumed was no different between fizzy and flat and no runner had to stop running due to GI symptoms.

In conclusion, if you prefer drinking carbonated drinks on the move and find the bubbles don't upset your stomach, then go ahead – but they won't give you any advantage over flat drinks. If its cola you crave, dilute it one or two parts to one part water to give you a better carb-concentration (4–8 per cent) for maximum absorption. Bear in mind that it is a very acidic drink with the ability to dissolve tooth enamel – so swish water around your mouth afterwards. Better still, opt for plain water during runs less than 60 minutes or orange juice diluted with equal amounts of water for a 4–8 per cent carbohydrate drink naturally packed with vitamins and minerals.

Why have carbohydrates during exercise?

Studies have shown that consuming carbohydrates, whether in liquid or solid form, during workouts lasting over 60 minutes can help you keep going longer. You will top-up blood sugar levels and fuel your muscles, particularly in the latter stages of your workout when glycogen reserves are likely to be low.

However, extra carbohydrates do not provide performance benefit during workouts lasting less than 60 minutes.

How much carbohydrate during exercise?

To give your muscles a decent carbohydrate boost during exercise, particularly in the final glycogen-depleted stages, you need to take in at least 30 g of carbohydrates per hour during your workout. Researchers at the University of Texas in Austin recommend 30–60 g per hour, depending on your body weight (heavier exercisers need more) and exercise intensity (more for harder workouts). That's equivalent to about 120–240 calories of carbohydrates per hour. There is no value in consuming more than 60 g as the muscles cannot use it.

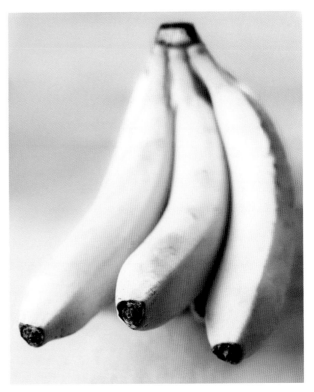

What to consume?

Choose fast-burning carbohydrates, such as drinks and foods with a high or moderate GI, as you need to get the carbohydrate into your bloodstream rapidly. Sports drinks, energy gels and energy bars are suitable as they are virtually pure carbohydrate (glucose, sucrose and maltodextrin) but more traditional foods such as bananas, fruit bars, cereal or breakfast bars (without hydrogenated fats), low-fat biscuits (e.g. fig rolls), malt loaf, dried fruit and chocolate work equally well. If you prefer savoury options, try rolls, bagels, sandwiches, rice cakes and crackers. Choose products containing less than 5 g fat per portion.

Which carbohydrates work best: liquid or solid?

Whether you choose solid or liquid carbohydrates makes no difference to your performance, provided you drink enough water. For most actitivities liquid carbohydrates are the most practical option. They provide vital fluid, quench your thirst and deliver a fixed concentration of carbohydrates so you know how much you are getting.

But carrying a sports drink with you on a long run, for example, is not always easy. It is heavy and can slow you down in a race. Solid carbohydrates have the advantage of being considerably lighter – just make sure you can get water somewhere en route. Do not skimp on your usual drink volume otherwise you will end up with a concentrated goo sitting in your stomach.

If you decide to take solid food it needs to be portable, palatable, non-perishable and very easy to eat. *See* 'What to consume?' (page 53) for suggestions for easy workout foods. Experiment to find the best drinks and foods for you.

How often should you consume carbohydrate?

Start consuming carbohydrate early in your workout, ideally in the first 30 minutes. It takes at least this time for the carbohydrate to reach your muscles and for the energy boost to kick in, so don't wait until you feel tired.

Your goal is to maintain a steady supply of carbohydrate entering your bloodstream. Aim to consume 15–30 g every 15–30 minutes. That is equivalent to half an energy gel pouch, one banana or half a 15 g bar of chocolate.

Won't the extra carbohydrates stop you from losing weight?

If you're exercising to lose weight, opt for plain water instead of sports drinks. Carbohydrate-rich drinks, gels and bars all add extra calories to your daily tally and may even supply as many – or more – calories as you are burning off! If you are training hard for longer than 60 minutes, choose a more dilute drink (e.g. one part juice to two parts water) and ensure you count the calories as part of your total daily intake.

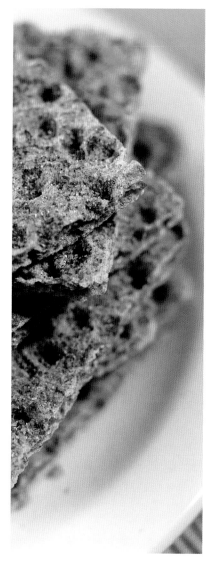

CARB UP FOR BETTER IMMUNITY

Does intense training often leave you susceptible to colds and infections? It is ironic that moderate training boosts your immune system but hard training can lower your defences against germs and viruses – especially when combined with poor eating habits. The reason? Heavy prolonged training results in increased levels of stress hormones (e.g. adrenaline and cortisol), which inhibits your immune system. Do not despair. Researchers from the University of Birmingham suggest the following:

- Ensure you eat enough calories to match your needs – remember to eat more on the days you train.

- Ensure you are consuming plenty of foods rich in immunity-boosting nutrients – vitamins A, C, E, and B6, zinc, iron and magnesium. Best sources are fresh fruit, vegetables, whole grains, beans, lentils, nuts and seeds.

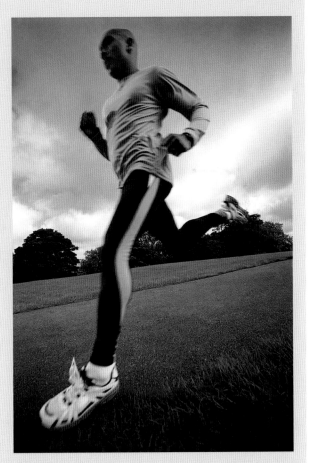

- A modest antioxidant supplement may help to boost your defences and reduce the risk of upper-respiratory infections (*see* page 98). Avoid mega-doses.

- Avoid training in a carbohydrate-depleted state, e.g. following a low-carbohydrate diet. Low glycogen stores are associated with increases in cortisol levels and suppression of your immune cells.

- During long tough workouts, consume 30–60 g of carbohydrate per hour to stave off the rise in stress hormones and the associated drop in immunity.

- Drink plenty of fluid. This increases your saliva production, which contains anti-bacterial proteins that can fight off air-borne germs.

- Try taking supplements of echinacea for up to 4 weeks during a period of hard training. Studies with athletes and non-athletes have shown that echinacea boosts the body's own production of immune cells and results in greater protection against minor illnesses.

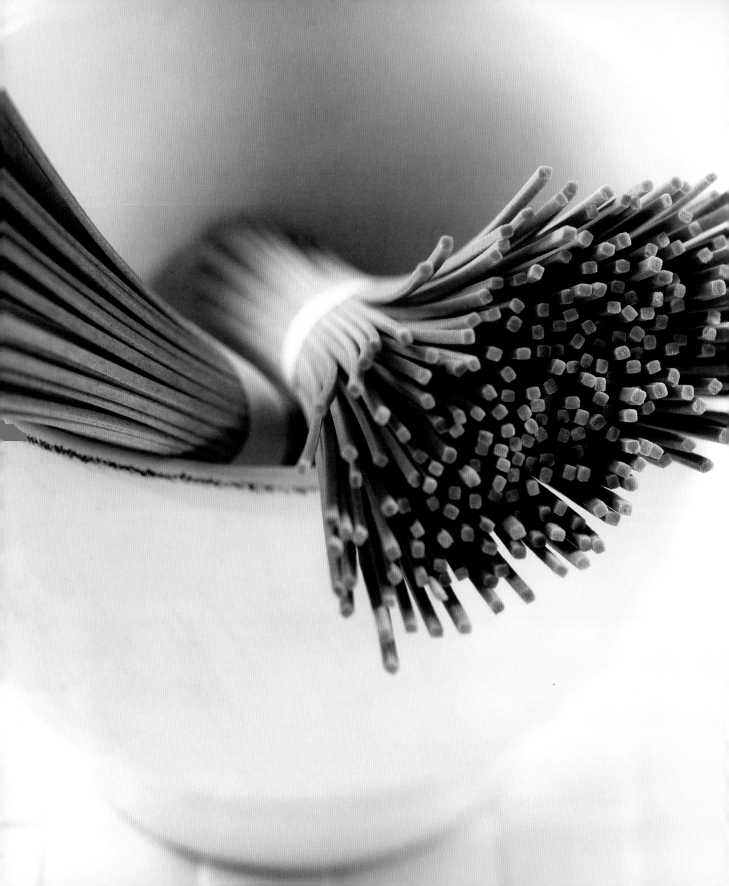

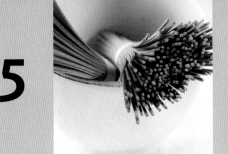

5 after training

The quicker you can begin refuelling after exercise, the quicker your body will recover. Any workout depletes your stores of glycogen – the readily available fuel stored in your muscles – and breaks down muscle tissue. Your aim is to rebuild these fuel stores and repair damaged muscle fibres as soon as possible. It is during this post-exercise period that your body gets stronger and fitter. Wait too long and you'll feel sluggish; get it right and you'll recover faster. Follow the practical steps outlined in this chapter and you will be well on the road to recovery.

Replacing lost fluids

How much to drink?

Start drinking before you even get showered and changed. The sooner you begin replacing the fluid you have lost through sweat, the sooner you will recover and cut the risk of post-workout dehydration. Fail to drink enough and you will feel listless with a risk of headache and nausea. As a rule of thumb, you need to drink 750 ml of water for every 0.5 kg of body weight lost during your workout. (1 kilogram of lost weight is equal to 1 litre of sweat, which needs to be replaced with 1.5 litres of fluid). Try to drink around 500 ml over the first 30 minutes, little and often, then keep sipping until you are passing clear or pale urine. Drinking slowly rather than guzzling the lot in one go will hydrate you better. If you pass only a small volume of dark yellow urine, or if you feel headachy and nauseous, then you need to keep on drinking.

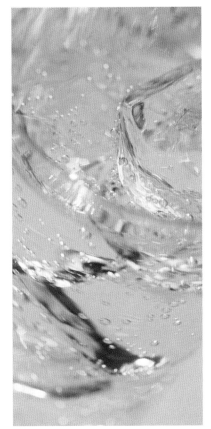

What to drink?

If you have exercised for less than an hour, plain water is a good choice followed by a carbohydrate-rich snack within 2 hours. For longer or particularly intense workouts, a drink containing carbohydrate (sugar or maltodextrin) and sodium may further speed your recovery. According to research at the University of Iowa, carbohydrate at levels of approximately 6 g carbohydrate per 100 ml increases the speed of water absorption into the bloodstream. Try fruit juice diluted with an equal volume of water, diluted squash (1 part squash: 6 parts water) or an isotonic sports drink containing 3–8 g carbohydrate per 100 ml. 'High energy' or 'recovery' drinks contain higher levels of carbohydrate: up to 12 g per 100 ml, mostly in the form of maltodextrin. These drinks may be useful following intense workouts longer than 90 minutes and are popular with ultra-endurance athletes.

Avoid refuelling after exercise with an alcoholic drink. Rehydrate with water or a sports drink before celebrating with lager, beer or shandy (the extra fluid will help attenuate dehydration) or alternate water with an alcoholic drink.

Reloading muscle glycogen

When to eat or drink?

Whether you are hungry or not, the quicker you consume food or drink after a workout, the quicker your body will recover. The enzymes that are responsible for making glycogen are most active immediately after your workout, leaving you a 2-hour window to reload your muscle glycogen. Carbohydrate is converted into glycogen one and a half times faster than normal during this post-exercise period. Wait more than two hours and your body's ability to convert what you eat or drink to glycogen drops by 66 per cent. The longer you wait, the longer it will take to start the recovery process.

If you work out daily, speedy recovery is crucial so have a carbohydrate-rich drink or snack (*see* page 61) as soon as possible after your workout – ideally within 30 minutes and no later than 2 hours.

GET YOUR ANTIOXIDANTS

Have you noticed how, after vigorous training, your muscles sometimes felt really sore? One of the factors responsible is the build-up of free radicals (molecules that have one or more unpaired electrons in their orbit) generated during exercise. In the short term, free radicals can damage cell membranes and make the muscles sore. While regular exercise increases the body's natural defences against free radicals, you can boost them further by consuming plenty of foods rich in antioxidant nutrients. Antioxidants are found in fruits, vegetables, whole grains and pulses.

Q&A

Question: *Should I eat a salty snack after exercise to replace lost sweat?*

Answer: Consuming extra sodium (salt) post-exercise is unnecessary and, in most cases, unadvisable. The sodium lost in sweat is a relatively small amount, even in hot weather, and is easily replaced by your usual diet. However, you may benefit from a sports drink containing low levels of sodium (around 0.5–0.7 g per litre) if you have been sweating heavily, for example, after hard exercise longer than an hour. The purpose of the sodium is to help your body retain water and to reduce urine output, thus encouraging rehydration (large volumes of any fluid promote urination as blood levels of sodium are temporarily diluted). Sodium will also make you feel thirstier, thereby causing you to drink more. But check the sodium content of the drink and make sure you count this towards your daily intake.

What to eat?

Begin refilling glycogen stores with a high-carbohydrate snack, aiming to consume 1 gram of carbohydrate per kilogram of bodyweight; for instance, a person weighing 70 kg needs to consume 70 g of carbohydrate. It doesn't matter whether you consume solid food or liquid nutrition – eat or drink whatever feels right (*see* page 61 for suggestions). Including a little protein with the carbohydrate will speed glycogen recovery further. The combination of carbohydrate and protein stimulates insulin release, which prompts the muscle cells to take up glucose and amino acids from the bloodstream. It also minimises protein breakdown and encourages muscle rebuilding.

Studies at the University of Texas at Austin, United States, have found that a ratio of about 3 parts carbohydrate to 1 part protein boosts glycogen storage by almost 40 per cent. It also promotes faster muscle repair and growth in weight trainers. US researchers have also shown that protein with carbohydrate reduces post-exercise muscle soreness.

So, your post-workout meal or snack should, ideally, comprise 20–25 g protein and 60–70 g carbohydrate.

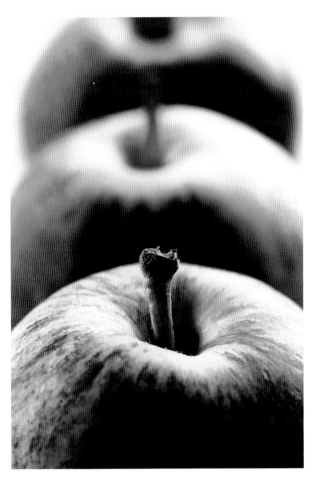

High or low GI after exercise?

Immediately after exercise, opt for a moderate- to high-GI snack or drink to deliver carbohydrate to your fuel-depleted muscles. A combination of carbohydrate with a little protein during the 2-hour post-exercise period promotes faster insulin release and thus a faster uptake of glucose from the bloodstream by the muscle cells. Try rice cakes with peanut butter or a handful of dried fruit and nuts. The box 'Refuelling snacks' on page 61 gives further suggestions.

However, choose low GI meals thereafter. Researchers at Loughborough University have found that eating low GI meals during the 24 hours following exercise improves endurance during your next workout. What's more, it also encourages the body to burn more fat and less carbohydrate, which helps shed unwanted pounds as well as improve performance. (*See* the box 'Refuelling meals' on page 62.)

Q&A

Question: *If I don't feel hungry after training, should I force myself to eat?*

Answer: Ironically, hard endurance training, particularly in warm conditions, can sometimes suppress your post-workout appetite. This is because more of the blood flow is concerned with exercising muscles, so the hunger signals your brain receives from your gut sensors become weakened. If the thought of eating straight after a workout makes you feel queasy, try liquid meals such as smoothies, yoghurt drinks, flavoured milk, milkshakes or meal replacement (carbohydrate/protein) drinks. (See box 'Refuelling snacks' on page 61.)

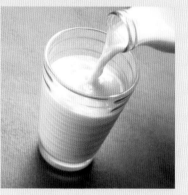

Q&A

Question: *Is it true that the calories I eat after a workout won't be stored as fat?*

Answer: Not exactly: while carbohydrate calories after exercise will be converted preferentially into glycogen, they can also be converted into fat if you consume too much. The enzymes that turn carbohydrates into glycogen in your muscles can only comfortably handle 50–70 g carbohydrate every 2 hours. Eat too much too soon and the resulting 'overspill' will be converted into fat. So, keep a check on portion sizes and opt for snacks and meals with a low glycaemic load (GL; see pages 7–8) such as yoghurt, a jacket potato with tuna or a cheese sandwich. Avoid meals or snacks with a high-GL and large portions of low-GI foods; for example, big bowls of pasta, jam sandwiches or even large volumes of energy drinks may give you more carbohydrate than you need.

REFUELLING SNACKS

(To be eaten within 2 hours after exercise.)

■ *A couple of pieces of fresh fruit with a glass of milk.* Fruits are a terrific natural source of low-GI carbohydrate as well as vitamin C and other antioxidants. They are easy to eat on the go – carry a supply with you during the day so you're never far from a healthy snack.

■ *1 or 2 cartons of yoghurt.* Fruit yoghurt contains almost the ideal carbohydrate to protein ratio (12:4 g per 100 ml) for speedy post-workout refuelling.

■ *A smoothie (crushed fresh fruit whizzed in a blender).* You can create your own flavour combinations but, in general, bananas, strawberries, pears, mango and pineapple give the best results. Add some yoghurt or milk for a protein boost.

■ *A home-made milkshake.* Use milk, yoghurt and fresh fruit (such as bananas and strawberries) for an excellent mixture of protein, carbohydrate and those all-important antioxidants.

■ *A yoghurt drink.* Pro-biotic yoghurt drinks are great for boosting immunity as well as supplying protein (3 g), carbohydrate (12 g) and calcium.

■ *Flavoured milk.* This was hailed as the perfect sports drink following a study published in the *International Journal of Sport Nutrition and Exercise Metabolism* (2006). The study showed that chocolate milk improved endurance more than conventional carbohydrate-only sports drinks because it contains the ideal ratio of carbohydrates to protein (14:4 g per 100 ml) to help refuel tired muscles.

■ *A sports bar.* Bars containing a mixture of carbohydrate and protein are handy after workouts.

■ *A tuna or cottage cheese sandwich.* Any kind of low-fat protein food together with some kind of (preferably wholemeal) bread – whether sliced, rolls, bagels, pitta or wraps – makes a great refuelling snack.

■ *A handful of dried fruit and nuts.* Dried fruits not only provide carbohydrate but also vitamins, minerals, antioxidants and fibre. Although nuts contain fat it is the healthy, unsaturated kind.

■ *A few rice cakes with jam and cottage cheese.* Rice cakes are a gym-goers' favourite – easy to carry around and munch while you're on the go. Just add a little protein for a well-balanced post-workout snack.

■ *A bowl of wholegrain cereal with milk.* Cereal and milk (or yoghurt) makes an easy breakfast after an early morning workout.

■ *A bowl of porridge made with milk.* Porridge is an ideal recovery food as it provides carbohydrate, protein, B-vitamins, iron and fibre. It has a low GI, gives a prolonged release of energy and should keep your muscles refuelled for a few hours.

■ *Jacket potato with tuna or cottage cheese.* Top your jacket potato with a low-fat high-protein food – try tuna, cottage cheese, chicken or baked beans – and add a side salad.

■ *A meal replacement (protein/carbohydrate) shake.* Shakes made up with milk or water are an easy and convenient mini-meal in a glass. Powders and ready-to-drink versions generally contain a balanced mixture of carbohydrate (usually as maltodextrin and sugar), protein (usually whey), vitamins and minerals.

Q&A

Question: *I work out in the evening and often don't return home until 9 or 10 o'clock. Should I eat anything at this late hour?*

Answer: Always eat and drink after your workout no matter how late it is. Your body needs carbohydrate, protein and other nutrients to replenish fuel stores and recover after training. Skipping that post-workout meal will delay recovery and leave you feeling sluggish the next day. Provided you don't over-eat, these calories will not be turned into fat.

To ensure you are properly fuelled before your evening workout, aim to consume the majority of your calories and nutrients during the early part of the day – have a good breakfast and lunch, with two or three balanced snacks in between meals. After working out, have a drink straightaway (water, diluted juice or a sports drink) then a light meal as soon as possible. Try a jacket potato with tuna or cottage cheese, pasta with a light sauce, chicken salad with rice, or baked beans and tomatoes on toast. Avoid weight gain by counting this meal towards your daily intake instead of additional to your usual daily meals. Plan ahead to ensure you have all the right foods and ingredients to hand. That way, you'll avoid the temptation of fast foods, sugary snacks or ready meals after your workout.

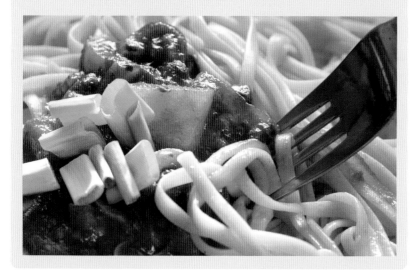

REFUELLING MEALS

- Pasta with tomato pasta sauce, grilled fish and salad
- Jacket potato, chicken breast baked in foil, broccoli and carrots
- Bean and vegetable hotpot with wholegrain bread
- Pitta bread, falafel and salad
- Rice with grilled turkey and steamed vegetables
- Lasagne or vegetable lasagne with salad
- Fish pie with cabbage and cauliflower
- Chilli or vegetarian chilli with rice and a green vegetable
- Dahl (lentils) with rice and vegetables
- Chicken curry with rice and vegetables
- Mashed or baked potato with grilled salmon and salad

Q&A

Question: *I feel ravenous after a workout – how can I avoid binge eating?*

Answer: An increased appetite is the body's way of telling you to eat. After a hard workout, you need to replace the fuel you have just used – but no more than that! It may be tempting to reward your workout efforts with an indulgent snack, but unless you keep a check on the calorie content, you may end up eating more than you've just burned off!

To prevent weight gain, opt for foods that give maximum volume per calorie to help satisfy your post-workout hunger and make you feel full for a long time. These foods will have a high water content, such as fresh fruits, salad and soup, a high fibre content, especially the soluble type (try beans on toast or lentil soup) or a viscous texture (such as porridge and potatoes). Including protein with carbohydrate in your post-workout snack or meal not only speeds glycogen recovery and muscle repair compared with eating carbohydrate alone, but also helps to satisfy your appetite and prevent overeating.

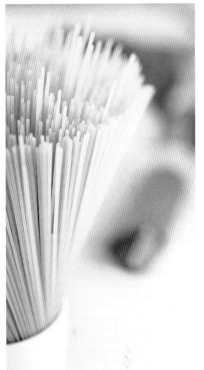

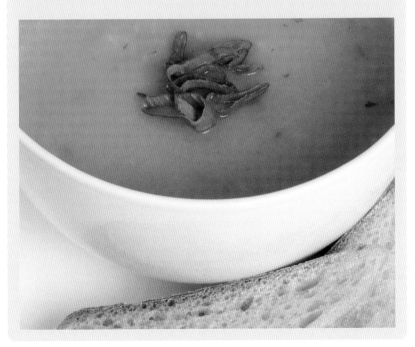

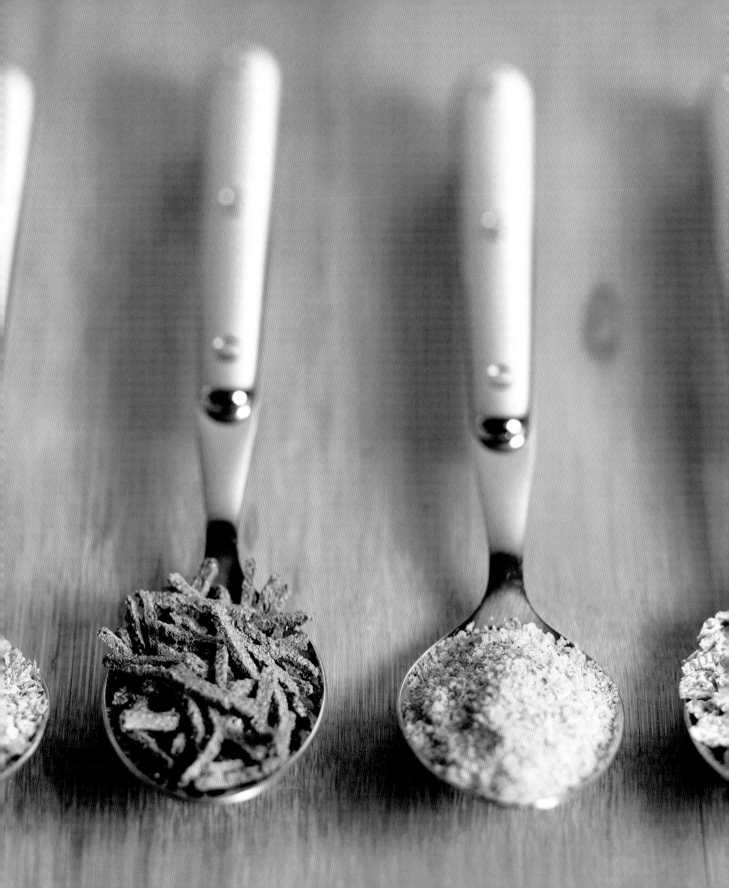

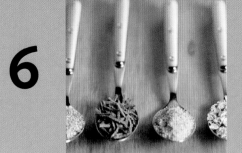

6 weight loss

When it comes to losing weight, those who exercise regularly have a head start. Whether you wish to lose a few pounds or have a bigger goal, exercise provides a healthy way to burn off extra calories. The problem is that even if you work out daily, it is hard to lose weight through exercise alone. Studies have shown that the secret to successful weight loss is regular exercise together with a healthy and careful calorie intake. Follow the eating tips throughout this chapter to help you drop those unwanted pounds.

How to lose weight?

The only proven way to lose weight is to eat fewer calories than your body uses as fuel for your activities. The idea is to find a diet and lifestyle that you can comfortably live with, rather than attempt to lose weight periodically with diets that are hard to maintain.

Don't diet

Many popular diets are based on gimmicks or unproven science and often involve cutting out certain food categories or limiting carbohydrates. They may help you lose weight in the short term but they are not sustainable. Most people don't like giving up favourite foods, whether chocolate, bread or cheese, so any diet that dramatically restricts these isn't likely to work in the long term. Sooner or later you'll give in to the temptation to eat the banned foods, thereby giving up the diet and putting the weight back on.

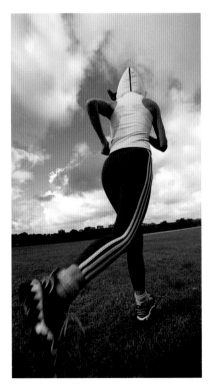

Long-term weight control is about making simple yet lasting changes to the way you eat and incorporating regular activity in to your daily schedule. Your eating plan should include all food groups – in particular, foods that:

■ satisfy your appetite

■ are high in complex and low-glycaemic carbohydrates

■ contain a modest amount of protein

■ have a high fibre and water content.

Do the calorie maths

Experts agree that 0.5–1.0 kg per week is a healthy and effective rate of weight loss. 0.5 kg of fat equates to roughly 3,500 calories. So, to lose 0.5 kg in a week you need to burn 3,500 calories more than you take in. This isn't as daunting as it sounds – lose 300 calories a day by foregoing two biscuits and drinking one less glass of wine and step up your expenditure by 200 calories a day, and you'll lose 0.5 kg a week.

HOW TO MEASURE PERCENTAGE BODY FAT

Percentage body fat is measured using skin-fold callipers or bioelectrical impedance. These techniques will tell you how much of you is muscle and how much is fat.

■ Skin-fold measurements using callipers are carried out by a trained person and measure the thickness of the layer of fat beneath the skin at various sites of the body. It works on the theory that 50 per cent of total body fat is stored under the skin. Most assessments involve measurements at four sites: the triceps, biceps, below the shoulder blades and mid-way between the hip and navel. The accuracy depends on the level of skill of the person taking the measurements. It is less accurate for very lean and obese individuals.

■ Bioelectrical impedance measures the resistance to a small electrical current passed through two points of the body. The more fat present, the greater the resistance. A person's hydration status and, for women, stage of menstrual cycle can affect the reading. It is also less accurate for very lean and very overweight individuals.

What is the secret to successful weight loss?

The secret ingredient in weight management is satiety, the feeling of fullness and satisfaction that you should have at the end of a meal. It may sound obvious, but the reason most diets fail is that they are too restrictive and don't satisfy hunger. To lose weight you need to be able to choose foods that are not only nutritious and enjoyable but also satisfy your hunger. If you don't feel

WHAT IS THE RIGHT PERCENTAGE OF BODY FAT?

You need body fat to survive: it is essential to the functioning of the brain, nerves and bone marrow, and it cushions the internal organs and keeps them warm. Women need a certain amount of body fat to maintain normal hormonal balance and menstrual function. All this accounts for about 3 per cent of bodyweight in men and 9–12 per cent of bodyweight in women. The remainder is stored under the skin and around the abdominal organs.

Scientists recommend body fat levels between 18 and 25 per cent for women and between 13 and 18 per cent for men. These ranges are associated with the lowest health risk in population studies. However, lower body fat levels are advantageous to performance in many sports: body fat levels in the region of 10–18 per cent in women and 5–10 per cent in men are common among elite athletes.

sated you will get hungry and tend to snack or overeat more readily. On the other hand, by eating mostly foods with a 'high satiety' rating, i.e. foods that are nutritious and also satisfy your hunger, you will find that you can feel full with fewer calories. **Feeling full and satisfied while eating foods you like makes it much easier to lose unwanted pounds.**

Why is satiety important?

Eating foods that satisfy your hunger will mean that you consume fewer calories – it's that simple. Obesity researchers have found that people tend to eat the same weight of food every day, regardless of the calorie content. When the water content of a dish is increased or extra vegetables are added, people eat the same amount but with fewer calories – yet they feel just as full and satisfied. So, by choosing foods that have fewer calories but eating your usual weight of food, you will end up eating fewer calories. In other words, opt for foods with a low energy density most of the time and eat smaller portions of foods with a high energy density.

Your personal weight loss plan

Step 1: Set yourself a goal

To help you succeed at losing weight, set an achievable goal and reward your positive behaviour. A goal has to be personal, specific, realistic and measurable.

- **Personal** – you have to believe in and truly want to achieve your goal. For example, *'I know that losing weight will allow me to fit into my clothes more comfortably and make me feel more confident, so I will begin to eat more healthily and take more exercise.'*
- **Specific** – you need to clearly define what you want to achieve then prioritise steps, organise plans and establish a timescale for reaching your goal. For example, *'I will limit myself to one chocolate bar once a week, on Saturdays, and eat three portions of fruit each day in place of biscuits.'*
- **Realistic** – your goal has to be realistic and attainable for your body shape and lifestyle. For example, *'I will lose 3 kilograms in six weeks.'*
- **Measurable** – you need to state how you will know when you've reached your goal. Keeping a food diary and training log will help you monitor your progress and allow you to see whether you met the goal. For example, *'I will eat five portions of fruit and vegetables each day of the week, as confirmed by my food diary.'*

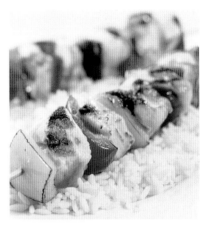

WHAT IS THE SATIETY INDEX?

Experts at the University of Sydney in Australia have developed a satiety index (SI) or 'fullness factor' to help people select foods for effective weight control. This is a measure of how long the consumption of a particular food will stop you feeling hungry again. SI is based on the energy density of food (ie. the number of calories per gram of food) as well as its fibre, water, fat and protein content. In general, foods with a high water and fibre content and a low fat content, such as fruits and vegetables, will fill you up more quickly than, for example, cheese and crisps.

See box on page 68 for the satiety index of some popular foods; the greater the number, the more filling the food is per calorie.

- *Agreed* – agree your goal with someone else and write it down. This signals a commitment to change and makes it more likely that you will be successful.
- *Reward yourself* – rewarding yourself when you have reached a goal helps you stay motivated and focused. Rewards can be something simple like a star for reaching a weekly target or something tangible like a new pair of shoes, a CD, a theatre trip or a beauty treatment.

Step 2: Visualise success

Visualise yourself looking slimmer. Draw a clear mental picture of how you will look and feel once you have achieved your goal. Focus hard on this image, including your face, body, clothes, hairstyle and as many colours and sounds as possible to help bring the image to life. Try to see yourself smiling, talking and moving around. Using visualisation in this way to persuade yourself that you are slim will give your body the message that being slim is a good thing. Very soon you will begin to eat healthier foods, become more active and achieve your weight loss goal.

Step 3: Get an idea of how many calories you should be eating

To lose weight, reduce your daily calorie intake by 15 per cent (multiply by 0.85). This will produce a calorie deficit of approximately 3,500 calories resulting in a fat loss of about 0.5 kg per week. (*See* 'How many calories do I need?' on page 2 to calculate your daily calorie needs.)

Step 4: Step up your physical activity

Increasing physical activity is an important part of your weight loss programme. For the best fat-burning results, make sure you include both resistance exercise and cardiovascular (endurance or aerobic) exercise in your weekly schedule. The American College of Sports Medicine recommends two weight training sessions a week in addition to three 20–40 minute sessions of aerobic activity.

SATIETY INDEX FOR SOME POPULAR FOODS	
Watermelon	4.5
Grapefruit	4.0
Carrots	3.8
Oranges	3.5
Fish	3.4
Chicken breast	3.3
Apples	3.3
Sirloin steak	3.2
Oatmeal	3.0
Popcorn	2.9
Baked potato	2.5
Low-fat yoghurt	2.5
Banana	2.5
Macaroni cheese	2.5
Brown rice	2.3
Spaghetti	2.2
White rice	2.1
Pizza	2.1
Peanuts	2.0
Ice cream	1.8
White bread	1.8
Raisins	1.6
Snickers bar	1.5
Honey	1.4
Sugar (sucrose)	1.3
Glucose	1.3
Potato crisps	1.2
Butter	0.5

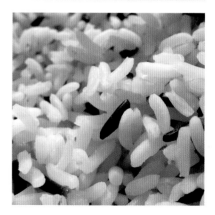

Resistance training

The most effective strategy for building or toning muscles and burning fat simultaneously is resistance or weight training. Muscle cells are up to eight times more metabolically active than fat cells, so the more muscle you have, the more calories you burn during daily activities. This doesn't necessarily mean lifting heavy weights – conditioning exercises using light or moderate weights tone muscle and prevents the loss of lean body tissue during weight loss. In general, train each muscle group for 2–4 sets of exercises with a weight you can lift only 8–12 times, taking 30 seconds' rest between sets. (See Anita Bean's *Six Week Workout* series, comprising *Better Body, Fab Abs, and Lovely Legs* (A & C Black, 2005) for an effective weights workout programme.)

You won't necessarily burn more calories lifting weights than doing aerobic exercise, but the increased muscle mass you develop as a result will make your body burn more calories every day. For every 0.5 kg of muscle gained through exercise, your metabolic rate increases by 30–40 calories a day. That's equivalent to an extra 1,200 calories a month or a further 0.5 kg fat loss over 3 months.

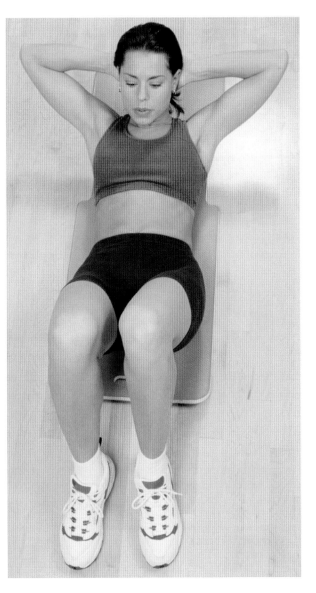

Q&A

Question: *Which burns more calories: weights or cardiovascular training?*

Answer: Both workouts burn a similar number of calories. However, according to a study at Colorado State University in the United States, one hour of weights workout increases the post-exercise calorie burn and metabolic rate considerably more than one hour of cardiovascular workout, the biggest difference occurring during the first two hours post-exercise. Furthermore, the study found that the metabolic rate of those who completed the weights workout remained higher than normal up to 14 hours later. So, intense weights workouts are the best way to boost your metabolic rate and burn more calories in the long term.

Cardiovascular exercise

Cardiovascular exercise burns calories and increases the body's ability to burn fat. It is any kind of activity that uses the large muscle groups of the body and can be kept up for 20–40 minutes, with your heart rate in your target training range count (*see* box on page 71). Try running, elliptical training machines, swimming, cycling, fast walking and group exercise classes. Vary your activities so you don't become bored. Remember, the higher the resistance, the more muscle you will build, so high-resistance activities such as rowing, stair-climbing, incline running and hard cycling are good for strengthening as well as defining muscles. Aim for 20–40 minutes per session, 3–5 times per week, but don't overdo it. Studies have shown that after about 60–90 minutes of aerobic activity, the body begins to break down and use muscle tissue as fuel; on a calorie-restricted diet, this happens earlier in your workout. Your basal metabolic rate (BMR) also slows, so you won't burn as many calories.

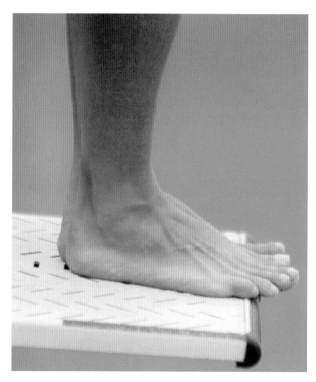

Q&A

Question: *Which is best for weight loss: high- or low-intensity exercise?*

Answer: High-intensity cardiovascular exercise, such as running, burns more body fat than low-intensity activities, such as walking, because it burns more calories. It also conditions the heart and lungs better and encourages the body to burn more fat – and less carbohydrate – 24 hours a day.

However, interval training is even more effective for fat burning as well as cardiovascular fitness. Alternate very intense periods of work with lower-intensity periods during which you recover. Try one or two minutes of high intensity alternating with two minutes of recovery. A study at Quebec University in Canada found that interval training (90-second bursts at 95 per cent of maximum heart rate) burned three and a half times more body fat than steady-rate, moderate-intensity exercise.

Step 5: Keep a food diary

Keeping a food diary will give you a much clearer idea of where your calories are coming from. Write down everything that you eat and drink for three days (or longer if you can manage it), noting the portion weights and sizes. Try to be as accurate as possible, recording the weights of everything and remembering to write down each snack and drink. Be as honest as possible – include the handful of crisps, the biscuits while making tea, the pint of beer after work. You may be surprised how quickly the calories add up or how often you nibble. Now put your eating habits to the test by comparing your portions with the recommendations of the Fitness Food Pyramid (see page 28). Look at your food diary and identify the foods or drinks that really aren't helping your fat loss efforts. Work out which types of food you need to reduce or increase. Saturated and trans fats (*see* pages 12–14) are non-essential and provide no benefit for the body. Main culprits are likely to be calorie-dense low-fibre snacks: biscuits, puddings, crisps, ice cream, cakes and chocolate bars.

Step 6: Eat mostly foods with a low energy density

Energy density is the number of calories in a fixed weight of food (usually expressed as calories per gram). Thus, foods with a low energy density contain relatively few calories per gram. To reduce your calorie intake and feel full on fewer calories, select mostly foods with an energy density less than 1.5 (*see* box on page 72). Eat foods with higher energy densities less often or in smaller portions.

HOW TO CALCULATE YOUR TARGET HEART RATE

The harder you work the more calories you will use. As a guide you should be working at a minimum of 60 per cent of maximum heart rate (MHR). To calculate your MHR, subtract your age in years from 220 then multiply by 0.6. However, for faster improvements in your fitness, try to work nearer to 85 per cent of your MHR.

For example, for a 30-year-old athlete working at 60–85 per cent of his MHR, his target heart rate range is 114–162 beats per minute:

$$220 - 30 = 190$$
$$190 \times 0.6 = 114$$
$$190 \times 0.85 = 162$$

Working lower than 114 is not efficient for conditioning his heart and lungs or fat burning, and working higher than 162 will further condition the heart and lungs but will reduce the effectiveness of the fat-burning programme.

You can lower the energy density of a dish or meal by adding water-rich ingredients (water has an energy density of zero) such as vegetables, salad or fruits, or by cutting out some of the fat. By increasing the amount of vegetables and fruit in a meal you can have satisfying portions for relatively few calories.

The fat content is also important – fat is the most energy dense nutrient (9 kcal per gram compared with 4 kcal per gram in protein or carbohydrate) and is, therefore, easy to overeat. If you take out some of the fat from a meal you can eat a larger portion for the same calories. For example, if you use skimmed milk instead of whole milk for making a sauce, you will get nearly twice as much for the same calories.

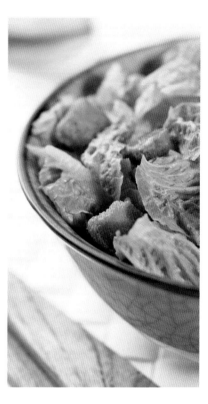

THE ENERGY DENSITY OF FOODS

Very low energy density (0–0.6) *Eat satisfying portions*	*Most fruits (e.g. strawberries, apples, oranges); non-starchy vegetables (e.g. carrots, broccoli); salad vegetables (e.g. lettuce, cucumber); skimmed milk; clear soups; fat-free or plain yoghurt*
Low energy density (0.6–1.5) *Eat satisfying or moderate portions*	*Bananas; starchy vegetables (e.g. sweetcorn, potatoes); low-fat plain/ fruit yoghurt; pulses (beans, lentils and peas); pasta, rice and other cooked grains; breakfast cereals with low-fat milk*
Medium energy density (1.5–4.0) *Eat moderate to small portions*	*Meat, poultry, cheeses, eggs, pizza, chips (fries), raisins, salad dressings, bread, ice cream, cake*
High energy density (4.0–9.0) *Eat small portions or substitute low-fat versions*	*Crackers, crisps, chocolate, sweets, croissants, biscuits, cereal bars, nuts, butter and oils*

Step 7: Choose fibre-rich foods

Eating more fibre-rich foods can help to reduce calorie intake. Fibre expands in the gut, thereby making you feel fuller and helping to prevent overeating. It also helps to satisfy your hunger by slowing the rate that foods pass through your digestive system and stabilising blood sugar levels. Studies have shown that people who increased their fibre intake for 4 months ate fewer calories and lost an average of 5 lb – with no dieting!

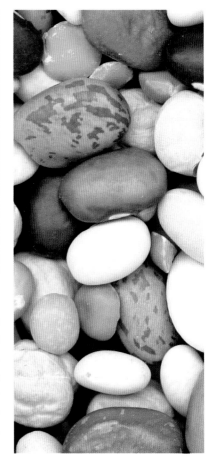

EATING FIBRE-RICH FOODS

■ Opt for breakfast cereals labelled wholegrain or oat-based cereals, for example, porridge, bran flakes, muesli or Shredded Wheat.

■ Swap white bread for wholegrain breads, such as wholemeal, rye and oatmeal, and eat wholegrain crackers and biscuits.

■ Use beans and lentils in one-pot dishes, soups, salads or stews and bulgur wheat in casseroles or stir-fries.

■ Eat at least five portions of fruit and vegetables each day and include at least one portion at each meal.

■ Add wholemeal flour or oatmeal when making cakes, muffins or fruit crumbles.

Step 8: Include lean protein

High-protein foods suppress the appetite longer and help prolong satiety more than foods high in carbohydrate or fat. Therefore, make sure you include adequate amounts of lean protein. Skipping protein may induce hunger. Include 2–4 portions (140–280 g) of high-protein foods (poultry, fish, low-fat dairy foods, beans, eggs, tofu) daily, depending on your fitness programme or sport. Daily, you should aim for 1.2–1.8 g of protein per kg of body weight; *see* also page 29). However, eating more protein than you need won't help you to lose weight faster, boost your metabolism or build muscle.

Step 9: Eat less fat

Reducing the amount of fat you consume lowers the energy density of your diet. This means you can eat bigger portions for the same or even fewer calories. But don't cut fat out of your diet completely – you need a certain amount of 'healthy' fats: the unsaturated fats found in fish, nuts, seeds and their oils (*see* page 29). Fats should provide around 20–25 per cent of calories consumed, with most coming from unsaturated sources. Cut down on foods rich in saturated and hydrogenated fats (butter, fatty meats, burgers, pastry, biscuits and cakes). Substitute reduced-fat or low-fat versions for high-fat foods (e.g. skimmed instead of whole milk). Use lower fat cooking methods (e.g. grilling instead of frying). Experiment with non-fat flavouring ingredients for your food, e.g. onions, garlic, lemon zest, herbs and spices.

Q&A

Question: *Will cutting more calories help me lose weight faster?*

Answer: Going on a strict diet may cause the pounds to drop off but can make you feel lethargic and weak, hindering your efforts in the gym. Worse still, your body can end up hoarding instead of burning fat. A sudden drop in calories sends a message to the body that starvation might be imminent, causing the body to conserve energy. As your body goes into survival mode, adapting to survive on a lower calorie intake, the rate at which you burn energy slows down. This means that when you stop dieting, you are likely to put the weight back on. To compensate for the low calorie intake, your body will start to break down muscle tissue for fuel. So, you can end up losing muscle as well as fat. *You should never cut your current calorie intake by more than 15 per cent*.

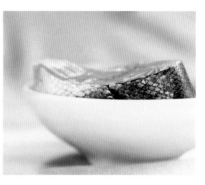

PLAN AHEAD

Plan your meals for the week. Sit down with a pen and paper and work out exactly what you need at the supermarket. Making a shopping list before you go shopping means that you're more likely to stick to it, and planning ahead means you won't get home from work tired and hungry only to discover there's nothing healthy in your fridge.

Twenty-two fat-loss tips that work

1: Eat several, smaller meals

Eating smaller meals more frequently not only reduces the chances of fat storage but also helps you recognise when you really are hungry. Spreading your meals more evenly through the day, as four to six small meals rather than two or three big ones, helps avoid blood sugar highs and lows and the resulting insulin surges. Insulin is a powerful anabolic hormone that drives glucose from the bloodstream into muscle cells and – when there's too much glucose – into your fat cells. Your aim should be to keep your blood glucose and insulin levels stable, so your body can manage them more easily. Eat regular snacks of fruit, nuts or seeds to give you slow-release energy throughout the day.

2: Limit your food choices

Research carried out at Tufts University in Massachusetts, United States, found that when people are presented with a wider variety of foods they eat considerably more. Also, when eating a single food, the individual's eating rate slows down, he or she is satiated more quickly and, therefore, he or she will eat less. The pleasure of eating a food increases up to the third or fourth bite then drops off. If you have lots of different foods on your plate you prolong the sensory pleasure, which stops you feeling full. The message here is to simplify your diet: place fewer types of food on your plate.

3: Practice portion control

It may sound obvious but larger portions make you eat more. Researchers at Cornell University, New York, found that people ate 33 per cent more food when given a large portion even when they disliked the food. Try putting smaller portions of foods with a high-energy density (such as meat, cheese and pizza) on your plate and larger portions of low-energy density foods such as vegetables on your plate. Check your portion sizes against those suggested in the Fitness Food Pyramid (*see* page 28).

4: Don't ban your favourite foods

Including your favourite foods in moderation will make your weight loss plan easier to stick to, if not pleasurable. If you know that you can eat a little of your favourite indulgence every day, you'll stop thinking of it as a forbidden food and then won't want to binge on it. So go ahead and include chocolate or ice cream in your nutrition plan but make sure it's only a little.

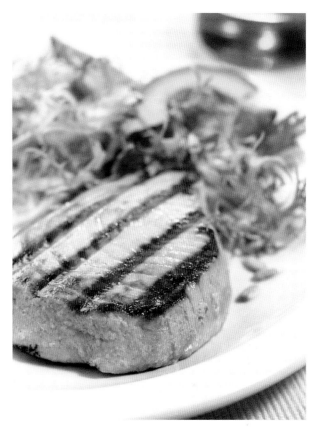

5: Don't skip breakfast

Starting the day with a healthy, filling breakfast dramatically increases your chances of eating healthily throughout the day. It also provides your body with fuel and kick-starts your metabolism, so you have the rest of the day to burn up those calories. The carbohydrates you eat at breakfast will be used to fuel your daily activities and workouts, instead of being stored as body fat (as they are if eaten in the evening).

If you don't eat breakfast, you are more likely to snack during the morning and overeat at lunch. Studies have shown that dieters who ate a high-fibre breakfast lost more weight than their breakfast-skipping counterparts and consumed 100–150 fewer calories for breakfast and lunch.

6: Start with salad

According to a 2004 study at Pennsylvania State University, United States, eating a large portion of low-energy density foods, such as salad or fruit, as a starter can cut the number of calories eaten during the main meal by 12 per cent. The fibre and water in the salad/ fruit takes the edge off the appetite, causing you to eat less of the higher calorie foods. (Take care not to add too much salad dressing.)

7: Sleep more

Sleeping an extra hour or so may help you lose weight, according to a study published in the journal *Sleep* in 2004. The study found that those who slept nine hours or more had, on average, a significantly lower body mass index than those who slept five hours or less. This is because lack of sleep boosts levels of the hormone ghrelin, which makes you feel hungry, while lowering levels of the hormone leptin, which makes you feel full. This hormonal imbalance sends a signal to the brain that more food is

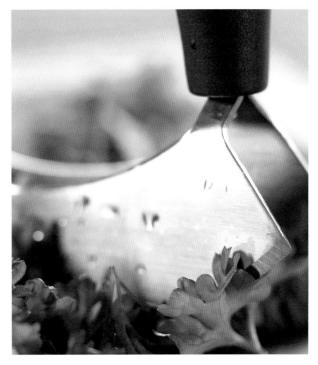

needed when, in fact, enough has been eaten. Research at the University of Chicago, United States, also shows that sleeping for four hours or less increases levels of another hormone, cortisol, which makes you feel hungry in the evening rather than sleepy.

8: Fill up with soup

Starting your meal with a bowl of chunky soup can cut your calorie intake by 20 per cent, according to a study by the University of Pennsylvania, United States. The idea is that fibre in soup fills you up so you'll eat less of the higher-calorie foods that follow. Avoid creamy soups, though: stick to vegetable varieties.

9: Switch off the TV

Don't eat in front of the television nor while you are working or reading – you are less likely to notice what you're eating. Studies have shown that the distraction of TV postpones the point at which people stop eating, with TV watchers eating approximately 12–15 per cent more than those who do not eat in front of the television. In addition, people who watch TV for more than four hours a day consume one-third more calories because they have more opportunity to nibble and less opportunity to exercise. Another study found that those who eat with family or friends consume up to 70 per cent more on average than those who eat alone. Social company, it seems, overrides satiety.

10: Distinguish between hunger and appetite

Unfortunately, it is easy to confuse hunger and appetite. Appetite is produced by external stimuli, such as the sight or smell of food or simply feeling bored. Real feelings of hunger are produced when blood sugar begins to fall. The difference is that appetite goes away when you distract yourself with another activity. Next time you feel the urge to eat, distract yourself by going for a walk, taking a bath or doing your nails. If you're still hungry then you know you need to eat.

11: Play music while you eat

Listening to music while you eat can help you lose weight. Studies have found that listening to relaxing music while eating makes you chew more slowly and eat less than when listening to frantic tunes.

12: Don't be 'fat phobic'

While cutting out high-fat foods will help you lose weight, don't completely cut fat out from your diet. This would be unhealthy and hinder your progress. Including foods rich in essential fats – oily fish, avocados, nuts, olives and seeds (*see* page 34) – in moderation can help burn body fat more efficiently, improve aerobic capacity and boost immunity. Fat also helps to give foods taste, so including it in moderation will help you stick to your eating plan. If you're eating 1,500 calories a day, aim to consume 33–42 g of healthy fats daily.

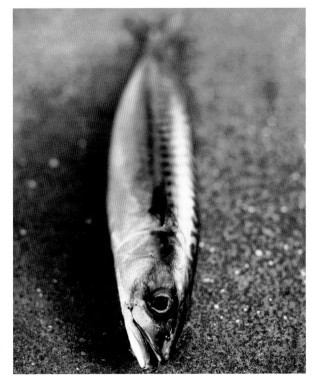

13: Eat slowly

You'll eat 15 per cent fewer calories if you sit down and take time to eat your meal rather than eating on the go. Studies have shows that people eat up to 15 per cent more calories when they rush at mealtimes. Scoffing your meal means that your hypothalamus – the part of the brain that senses when you are full – doesn't receive the right signals, which explains why you may feel hungrier sooner if you rush a meal.

14: Keep an eye on your alcohol consumption

Alcohol calories count too: if you enjoy several alcoholic drinks in an evening, they can sabotage your fat-loss plan. Alcohol calories can't be stored and have to be used as they are consumed – this means that calories excess to requirements from other foods get stored as fat instead. One small glass of red wine contains 85 calories and a bottle of lager contains 130 calories. If you have a drink, make sure you include it in your daily calorie allowance.

15: Drink water

Many people confuse thirst with hunger. Both thirst and hunger sensations are generated at the same time to indicate the brain's needs. If you don't recognise the sensation of thirst, you may assume that you are hungry and eat instead of drinking water. Next time you're feeling peckish, drink a glass of water and wait ten minutes to see if you are still hungry.

16: Eat fruit instead of drinking juice

Eating fruit is one of the best things you can do for your health; aim for 2–4 portions daily. However, you should only count a maximum of one portion of fruit juice towards your daily target. A glass of juice provides 120 calories but if you eat an orange instead (60 calories) you'll save 60 calories, consume more fibre and still get your daily vitamin C quota. Both fruit juice and dried fruit contain much higher concentrations of (natural) sugar than the fresh fruit they came from and are less satiating.

17: Beware of 'reduced-fat' labels

Eating foods labelled 'reduced-fat' may make you feel virtuous but it can trick your brain into letting you overeat. Many lower-fat versions of biscuits, ice cream, cakes and yoghurt contain extra sugar or modified starch in place of the fat, making their calorie count just as high. Unfortunately, the body is not very good at regulating the intake of high-calorie food, whether the calories come from fat or carbohydrate. You may keep eating, thinking you're being good, while actually you're being overloaded with calories. You would be better off eating the occasional biscuit or cake rather than regularly eating the reduced-fat versions.

18: Don't go shopping when you're hungry

If you go shopping when you're hungry you will be tempted to fill up your trolley with high calorie foods. Make a shopping list before you hit the supermarket – that way you'll avoid unplanned supermarket splurges in unhealthy foods. If you shop with a list you will be less likely to make impulsive food choices.

19: Replace half your carbohydrates with veggies

Try replacing half of your usual portion of carbohydrates (bread, pasta, potatoes) with vegetables such as carrots, broccoli, green beans or cauliflower. That way you won't feel like you're eating less.

20: Match every excuse to a solution

Do you snack on high-calorie foods during the day because you're always in a rush? The solution is to prepare meals in advance or, perhaps, to take a supply of healthy snacks with you to eat between meals. Do you always snack on high-calorie foods in front of the television? Eat an apple instead or, better still, think of an activity to take you away from the television.

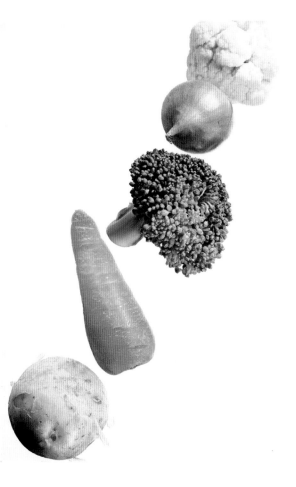

21: Carry healthy snacks

Always carry healthy snacks, such as apples, satsumas, nuts or small cereal bars, with you so you don't end up at the chocolate vending machine or snack food counter when you feel hungry.

22: Stock up with healthy foods

Keep a well-stocked supply of healthy foods that you love to make your fat-loss programme easy. Decide which new foods you're going to substitute for high-fat or sugary foods. This way, you'll keep yourself on track and avoid the temptation of slipping back into old eating habits. Remember, fruit, vegetables, pulses and wholegrain cereals give the best filling power for the minimum calories. They contain lots of water and fibre, which fill you up, slow down your eating speed and give best meal satisfaction. Choose the ones you like and stock up on those.

Six tips to boost your metabolism

1: Get moving

Up to two hours after vigorous exercise, you continue to burn calories faster than normal while your body replenishes its energy reserves and repairs muscle tissue. The longer and more intense your workout, the greater the 'after-burn'.

2: Tone up

To increase your metabolic rate in the long term, you have to add muscle. The American College of Sports Medicine recommends two weight training sessions a week: the increased muscle tone you develop as a result will make your body burn more calories every day.

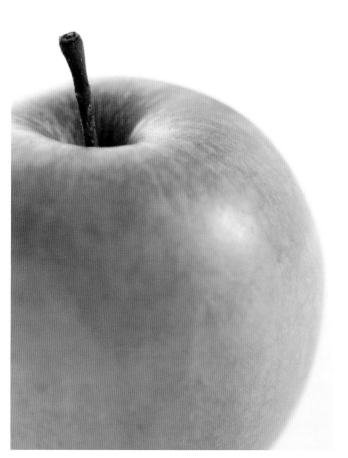

3: Eat small meals often through the day

Small, regular meals will keep your metabolism ticking over and are a much better way to burn off calories than, for example, one meal a day. Plan three meals and two or three snacks daily, spacing them out evenly. Your metabolism is boosted by about 10 per cent for two to three hours after you eat. Avoid skipping meals or leaving more than five hours between meals.

4: Eat enough protein

While eating in general raises your metabolic rate, protein boosts it the most: up to 20 per cent of a protein meal's calories may be burned off as heat.

5: Eat a healthy breakfast

Breakfast kick-starts your metabolism and allows you the whole day to burn off calories. A combination of carbohydrate and protein (for example, porridge made with semi-skimmed milk) will give you sustained energy.

6: Go for a walk after a meal

Moderate exercise, such as walking, after eating may increase your metabolic rate, turning more of the calories you have eaten into heat. Similarly, eating in the hour after vigorous exercise encourages food to be turned into energy rather than stored as fat, as the metabolic rate is also speeded up during this time.

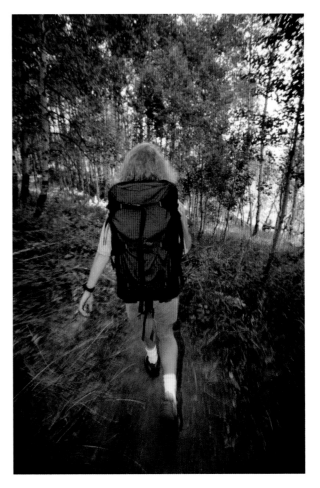

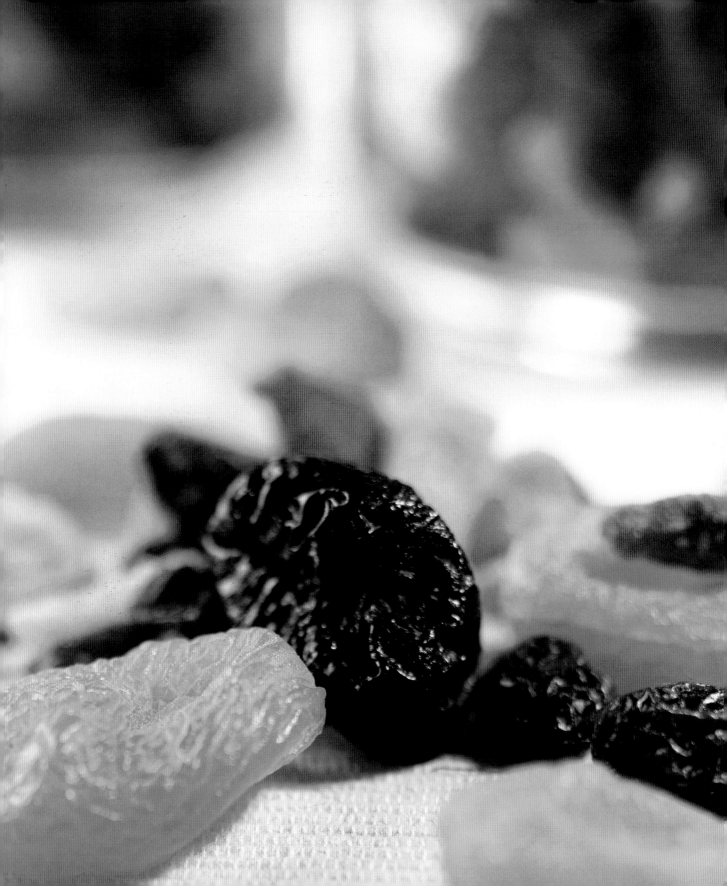

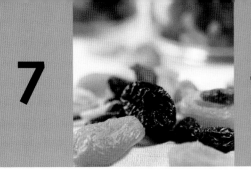

top 15 fitness foods

1: Bananas

Why they're good:

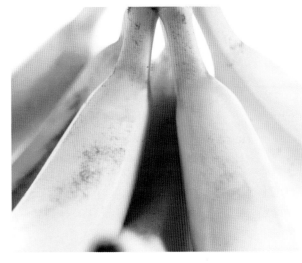

■ Bananas are cheap, portable and full of nutrients. An average banana provides around 90 calories and 15 g of carbohydrate from a mixture of three sugars (fructose, glucose and sucrose) and starch, which give it a moderate to low GI (52), although the GI increases with ripeness. Eating a banana will, therefore, produce a fairly slow rise in blood sugar, giving you a sustained energy supply.

■ The fibre in bananas is important for protecting against bowel cancer, lowering cholesterol and stabilising blood sugar levels.

■ Bananas also deliver potassium, which is essential for regulating fluid levels in cells, maintaining blood pressure and minimising the risk of stroke, and magnesium, which plays a key role in the formation of new cells and muscle contraction.

■ Bananas are a good source of vitamin B6, which is involved in the manufacture of red blood cells as well as the breakdown of proteins, carbohydrates and fats.

When they're good:

Bananas are best eaten 30–60 minutes before exercise, during workouts lasting more than an hour or right after training. Eat them on their own or blend with some milk or yoghurt for a nutritious smoothie.

2: Beans and pulses

Why they're good:

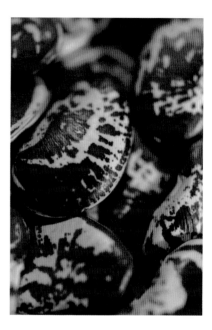

■ Beans have a very high satiety index (*see* pages 67–68), which means they digest slowly, fill you up and satisfy your hunger. They also have a low GI (26–48), which means a gradual increase in blood sugar and longer-lasting energy than most other foods.

■ Beans are a low-fat source of protein and are rich in the amino acid lysine, which is lacking in most other plant proteins. Eat with pasta, oats or rice to balance the amino acids of the meal and increase the overall protein quality.

■ Beans can help reduce the risk of heart disease. A study of 10,000 men and women found that those who ate beans or lentils at least four times a week had a 22 per cent lower risk of heart disease compared to those who ate them less than once a week. They also had lower blood pressure, blood cholesterol levels and a lower chance of diabetes.

■ The fibre in beans helps to keep 'bad' LDL cholesterol levels down while boosting 'good' HDL cholesterol.

■ Beans may help prevent cancer due to their high content of phytates and phytoestrogens (which have been linked to the prevention of breast cancer in particular).

■ Beans are rich in iron, which is essential for transporting oxygen around the body, as well as B-vitamins, zinc and magnesium.

When they're good:

Try to include beans or lentils in your main meals at least once a week, aiming to increase gradually to four times a week. According to a University of Sydney study, lentils eaten three hours before exercise may help increase your endurance significantly more than other carbohydrates.

3: Berries

Why they're good:

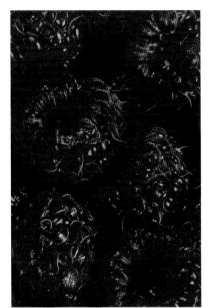

■ Berries are densely packed with vitamins and other phytonutrients. A US study ranked cranberries and blueberries at the top of the league table for antioxidant power, closely followed by blackberries, raspberries and strawberries. They contain compounds called *anthocyanins* – the pigment that gives berries their intense colour – that mop up damaging free radicals and help prevent cancer and heart disease.

■ Blueberries, raspberries and blackberries contain ellagic acid, another powerful antioxidant that fights cancer. Blueberries contain high levels of resveratrol, an antioxidant that helps combat free radicals.

■ Berries are rich in vitamin C, which, together with the anthocyanins, helps to strengthen blood capillaries and improve blood flow around the body.

■ Blueberries may help slow the ageing process, according to a study at the USDA Human Nutrition Centre on Ageing at Tufts University, USA.

■ Blueberries and cranberries have unique 'anti-stick' properties that help ward off urinary tract infections, ulcers and gum disease.

When they're good:

Eat at least three to four portions of fresh berries a week. If you can't get fresh berries, try dried blueberries or cranberries in muffins, bread and pancakes. They retain most of the antioxidant properties of fresh berries but contain less vitamin C.

4: Broccoli (and other green vegetables)

Why they're good:

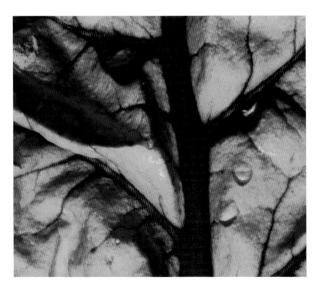

■ Broccoli and other cruciferous vegetables, such as Brussels sprouts, curly kale, cabbage, spinach and cauliflower, contain powerful antioxidants called sulforaphane and indoles, which disarm free radicals. Studies at Harvard Medical School and nearly 100 other studies have shown that eating broccoli may reduce the risk of certain cancers and heart disease. Just one daily serving (two broccoli florets) provides significant protection from cancers of the lungs, breast, stomach, colon and rectum.

- Green vegetables are rich in soluble fibre, which helps slow the absorption of carbohydrates from the intestines and promote stable blood sugar levels.

- Broccoli provides vitamin C and beta-carotene, two powerful antioxidant nutrients that stop the damage caused by free radicals. One serving (85 g) of cooked broccoli provides approximately 100 per cent of the recommended daily requirement of vitamin C.

- Brussels sprouts contain a compound called sinigrin (an isothiocyanate) which fights cancer by triggering pre-cancerous cells to die. Even one serving (nine sprouts) can have this effect!

When they're good:

Aim for five to seven portions of green vegetables per week. Choose broccoli that has tight, deeply coloured and dense florets; the deeper the colour, the more phytonutrients. When cooking broccoli, don't discard the stalk and leaves – they are rich in nutrients. Yellowing florets are a sign that the broccoli is old and has lost much of its goodness.

5: Breakfast bars

Why they're good:

- Breakfast cereal bars are convenient snacks for before, during or after training. They are made from cereal, sugars or syrup, and oil. They generally contain around 100 calories per bar, 2–5 g fat and 8–10 g sugar. The small portion size of most breakfast cereal bars also makes them a lower-calorie and low-fat alternative to chocolate and confectionery bars.

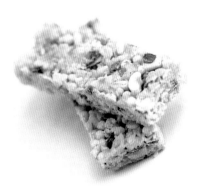

- Some popular brands contain harmful hydrogenated oils so check the ingredients list carefully.

- Many breakfast cereal bars are deceptively high in sugar, containing around one-third of their weight in the form of glucose syrup, fructose, invert sugar, sucrose or brown sugar (all different types of sugars), which gives them a high GI (around 70–75).

- The fibre content is generally low, with most supplying little more than 1 g of fibre per bar (around 5 per cent of a person's daily fibre requirement).

- On the plus side, most varieties contain added vitamins and minerals, which gives them the nutritional edge over chocolate bars and other energy bars.

When they're good:

Eat one when you need a quick boost of energy, for example, during workouts lasting longer than an hour or straight after training. Eating a breakfast cereal bar will boost blood sugar levels and kick-start glycogen re-fuelling.

6: Cereal bars

Why they're good:

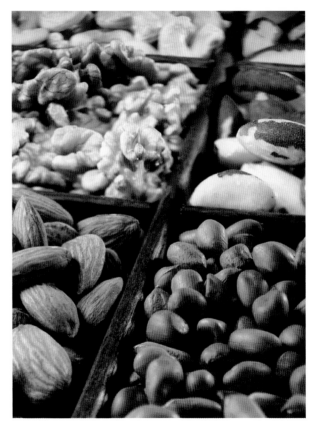

- Like breakfast bars, cereal bars are handy high-carbohydrate snacks that are lower in fat and higher in fibre than chocolate or confectionery bars. They are made from cereal grains, sugars, dried fruit, oil and various combinations of nuts, seeds, chocolate or yoghurt coating.

- Most bars provide between 120 and 180 calories but, as with breakfast bars, check the label carefully as many popular brands contain hydrogenated oil or fat as well as excessive amounts of sugar and glucose syrup.

- Choose bars that do not contain hydrogenated or palm oil and which list wholegrains (such as oats), dried fruit or nuts higher than sugars on their ingredients panel.

- Avoid 'yoghurt-coated' bars as the coating is mostly hydrogenated fats and sugar (not yoghurt!).

When they're good:

Cereal bars are useful when you have to eat on the move or refuel after training to replenish your glycogen stores.

7: Smoothies

Why they're good:

- Smoothies made with fresh fruit are a great way of meeting your five-a-day target for fruit and vegetables. They are packed with beta-carotene, vitamin C, phytonutrients and potassium.

- Smoothies are more nutritious than fruit juice because they contain all the fibre of the whole fruit.

- Make your own smoothie by whizzing fresh fruit (such as berries, bananas and pears) with a little fruit juice or yoghurt in a smoothie maker, liquidiser or using a hand-held blender. Add milk, ground almonds or a little omega-3 rich oil for extra nutrients.

- Check the ingredients of ready-bought versions – some brands contain minimal fruit and high levels of added sugar and artificial additives.

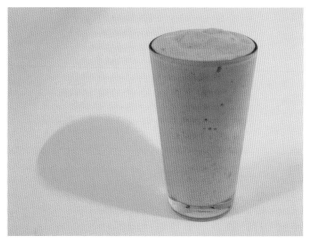

When they're good:

Smoothies are great for breakfast, as a snack on the go or as a refreshing post-workout drink.

8: Dried fruit

Why it's good:

- Dried fruit – raisins, sultanas, dried apricots, dried mangos, etc. – is a concentrated source of carbohydrate, which makes it a useful snack when you need a quick energy boost.

- As the fruit is dried, it provides concentrated fibre, potassium, phytonutrients and vitamins and minerals.

- According to a study at Tufts University, USA, apricots are rich in beta-carotene (five apricots provide one-sixth of a person's daily vitamin A needs) while prunes and raisins contain very high levels of antioxidants.

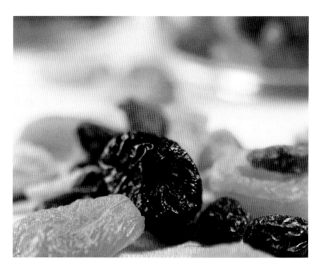

When it's good:

- Eat a handful of dried fruit after exercise (with water) to speed up glycogen refuelling.
- Try them on long cycle rides, but don't overdo it as the fibre content may upset your stomach.
- Dried fruit makes a handy snack for eating on the go.

9: Porridge

Why it's good:

- Porridge is a low-GI food, which means it provides sustained energy and boosts glycogen stores, with only a low risk of the carbohydrates turning into body fat.
- Consumed daily, oats can help lower cholesterol, thus preventing blood vessels furring up. They contain beta-glucan, a soluble fibre that mops up the precursors of cholesterol and whisks them out of the body.
- The fibre in oats makes you feel full relatively fast, stopping feelings of hunger. Thus porridge is filling and satisfying, with a high satiety index value (*see* pages 67–68).
- Oats are one of the few grains to contain high levels of vitamin E – a powerful antioxidant that helps protect the heart, reduces the risk of certain cancers, helps prevent premature ageing and mops up free radicals produced during intense exercise.
- According to a 2003 study published in the *American Journal of Clinical Nutrition*, including oats in your diet regularly will reduce the chances of developing Type-2 diabetes, because oats stabilise blood sugar levels.

When it's good:

- Porridge is ideal for breakfast or for eating 2–4 hours before a workout.

10: Nuts

Why they're good:

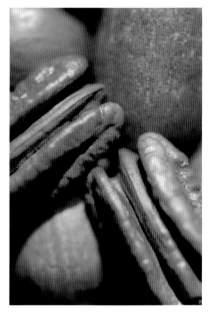

■ All nuts are a rich source of fibre, vitamin E (which helps keep the heart healthy), B-vitamins (which help release energy from food), folate (which lowers the risk of heart disease and helps prevent cancer) and magnesium (important for healthy bones and nerve and muscle function).

■ Almonds provide high amounts of calcium.

■ Peanuts are an excellent source of the antioxidant resveratrol (also found in red wine), which boosts your defences against cancer and heart disease.

■ Brazil nuts are a good source of selenium, a potent antioxidant that helps reduce signs of ageing, boosts the immune system and reduces the risk of cancer. One Brazil nut provides most of a person's daily requirement of this mineral.

■ Walnuts contain omega-3 oils, which not only lower blood cholesterol but also help promote post-exercise recovery.

■ Although nuts are high in fat (90 per cent of their calories come from fat), this is mainly the mono-unsaturated kind which guards against heart disease and lowers cholesterol levels. A US study found that people who ate 30 g of nuts at least five times a week were up to 51 per cent less likely to develop heart disease. A study at the University of Toronto, Canada, found that people who ate about 28 g of almonds (equivalent to a small handful) a day lowered their LDL ('bad') cholesterol levels by 4 per cent.

■ Nuts have a high satiety rating (*see* pages 67–68) – they satisfy hunger more readily than most other foods.

■ According to research at Purdue University in the USA, when eaten as part of a balanced diet, nuts can help with weight management. A study at Harvard Medical School in the USA found that people who ate nuts as part of a Mediterranean-style moderate-fat diet lost more weight and kept it off longer than those who followed a traditional low-fat diet. US researchers found that eating up to 85 g of peanuts a day lowered blood fat levels by up to 24 per cent without weight gain.

When they're good:

Eat nuts for a snack or add to cereals, homemade cakes, muffins and bars, yoghurt and salads. Have a handful of nuts with dried fruit after training to refuel glycogen stores and aid muscle repair. Choose unsalted varieties where possible; salted nuts encourage overeating.

11: Rice cakes with peanut butter

Why they're good:

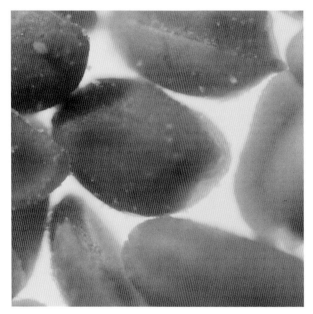

- Rice cakes provide high-GI (fast-absorbed) carbohydrate so, on their own, are good for boosting blood sugar levels immediately after training.

- Adding peanut butter (low GI) makes this snack even more effective for glycogen refuelling because you mix carbohydrate, protein and fat – which slows down the absorption of carbohydrates, lowers the GI and gives longer-lasting energy. It also tastes good!

- Peanut butter contains protein, fibre, heart-healthy monounsaturated oils and vitamin E.

- Also try rice cakes with avocado or guacamole (avocado dip), hummus (chickpea dip), cheese or low-fat soft cheese for a nutritious snack.

- Spread rice cakes with jam for a high-GI snack, for example, immediately after training, but don't eat too many otherwise the glycaemic load (GL) may be too high (*see* pages 7–8).

When they're good:

- As a quick nutritious snack.

- Good for eating 30 minutes before training or immediately afterwards for a blood-sugar boost and rapid glycogen replenishment.

- Don't overdo the peanut butter because of its fat content – limit yourself to about 3 tablespoons a day.

12: Salmon

Why it's good:

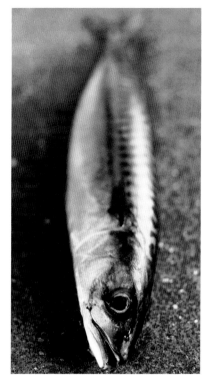

- Like other oily fish, salmon is a rich source of protein, vitamin A (needed for healthy eyes, skin and hair), vitamin D (needed to form strong bones and teeth) and the long-chain omega-3 fatty acids – eicosapentanoic acid (EPA) and docosahexanoic acid (DHA). It's also a good source of copper, zinc, vitamin E and selenium.

- Omega-3 fats reduce the risk of heart attack and stroke, lower blood fat levels and reduce the stickiness of platelets in the blood. The Multiple Risk Factor Intervention Trial, carried out in the USA, found that people who ate modest amounts of oily fish had a 40 per cent lower risk of death compared with other diets. Another study at the Harvard School of Public Health in the USA found that those who ate five or more servings of fish a week had one-third the risk of having a stroke compared to those who ate fish once a month or less.

- Omega-3 fats can alleviate inflammatory conditions, such as rheumatoid arthritis and joint stiffness or pain after hard exercise. They may also benefit your aerobic workouts by promoting better oxygen delivery to your muscles, reducing blood viscosity and make red blood cell membranes more flexible.

When it's good:

- Try to eat at least one portion (140 g) of salmon or other oily fish a week. Try herrings, sardines, fresh tuna, trout, pilchards and mackerel.

- Choose wild salmon to minimise any potential risk from dioxins and PCBs. Look for the words 'wild pacific' or 'Alaska' on fresh and frozen fillets or 'Alaska salmon' on the lid of tinned salmon.

13: Dark chocolate

Why it's good:

- Dark chocolate (with 70 per cent cocoa solids) contains useful amounts of magnesium, copper and iron as well as antioxidant flavanoids.

- Tests at Kings College in London have shown that dark chocolate has the same antioxidant activity as fruit and vegetables.

■ Research at the University of California found that the flavanoids in dark chocolate may lower heart disease risk, and a 2006 Dutch study showed that dark chocolate might also lower blood pressure.

■ These benefits only apply to dark chocolate, not milk chocolate, which contains less than half the levels of flavanoids found in dark chocolate. Also, adding milk to chocolate or even drinking a glass of milk at the same time as eating dark chocolate dilutes their effect severely. A study at the University of Glasgow found that dark chocolate boosted levels of antioxidants in the bloodstream by 20 per cent for 4 hours but milk chocolate or dark chocolate eaten with a glass of milk did not.

■ Check the label for 'vegetable fat'. Many popular brands of chocolate made in the UK contain it – it is hydrogenated fat, a source of trans fats (*see* pages 13–14) which are linked to heart disease.

■ Opt for plain chocolate rather than 'filled chocolate' bars containing caramel or nougat. An average 'filled' bar contains up to 18 per cent saturated fat.

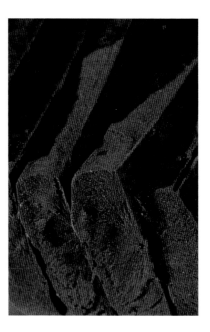

When it's good

There is nothing wrong with enjoying chocolate (especially dark chocolate) from time to time as an indulgent treat. Scientists at the University of Bath found that 70 per cent of people who ate chocolate regularly said they felt happy compared with just 41 per cent of those who ate no chocolate at all. A small (40 g) bar, eaten slowly and savoured, will add a smaller calorie and fat load (204 calories; 11.5 g) than, for instance, a bag (116 g) of chips (400 calories; 16 g).

14: Wholegrain breads and cereals

Why they're good:

■ An international research review published in 2005 found that people who regularly eat wholegrain foods have a 20–40 per cent lower risk of heart disease and stroke compared with those who rarely eat wholegrain foods. Just four servings of wholegrains (such as wholewheat bread, wholegrain breakfast cereals, wholemeal pasta, brown rice, millet and barley) give the same blood-cholesterol-lowering benefits as 'statin' drugs.

Wholegrains provide both insoluble and soluble fibre. Insoluble fibre promotes a healthy digestive system and lowers the risk of bowel cancer. Soluble fibre helps lower blood cholesterol levels and reduces the risk of heart disease. A US study published in the medical journal *Circulation* concluded that adding 3 g of soluble oat fibre to your daily diet lowers 'bad' LDL cholesterol by 10 per cent. A 2004 US study involving 330,000 adults concluded that for every 10 g of cereal fibre consumed a day (equivalent to three slices of wholegrain bread), the risk of death from heart disease was cut by 25 per cent. They also found a 27 per cent decrease in the risk of dying from heart disease. The US dietary guidelines recommend a minimum three servings of wholegrain foods (equivalent to three slices of wholemeal bread) a day.

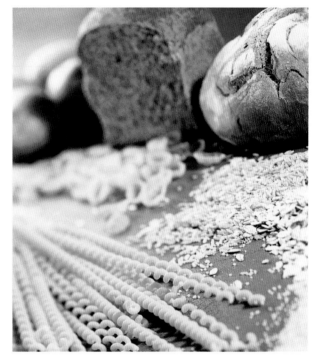

Wholegrains help lower the risk of colon cancer. They contain phytic acid, which decreases the rate at which cancer cells spread, and enhances the immune system.

Wholegrains contain many phytonutrients, important in illness prevention. For example, wheat contains lutein, zeaxanthin and beta-cryptoxanthin, potent antioxidants that protect against cancer.

Wholegrains are good sources of iron (which transports oxygen to muscle cells), zinc (for making new cells, healing and fighting infection), vitamin E (which strengthens the immune system) and selenium (which helps mop up free radicals).

When they're good

Aim for at least three portions of wholegrains daily. These can include wholewheat bread, wholegrain breakfast cereals, wholemeal pasta, brown rice, millet, barley, quinoa, rye and corn.

Look for the words 'wholemeal' or 'wholegrain' on labels. 'Wheatgerm' or 'brown' do not mean wholegrain; such products are generally refined versions with added wheatgerm or bran.

15: Yoghurt

Why it's good:

■ Yoghurt is low in fat and a rich source of protein, calcium and B-vitamins. It has a high satiety index (*see* pages 67–68).

■ Fruit yoghurt contains a near-perfect combination of carbohydrate (lactose, or milk sugar, and sucrose) and protein for post-workout recovery. University of Texas researchers found that a ratio of 3:1 accelerates glycogen storage post-workout. One pot of yoghurt provides almost one-third of the daily requirement of calcium (200 mg) as well as a healthy dose of B-vitamins (which help release the energy from carbohydrates).

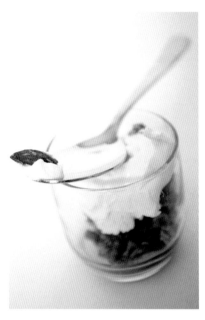

■ Foods high in calcium can trick the body into working overtime and shedding weight, according to a study at the University of Tennessee, USA. Obese people who ate two cartons of low-fat yoghurt a day but who made no other changes to their eating habits over a year lost nearly 5 kg (11 lb.) more than those who were not given yoghurt. They also had a six-fold greater decrease in waist measurement. It is thought that getting enough calcium stimulates the body to burn fat and also reduces the new fat the body lays down. Keeping up your calcium intake will also help prevent osteoporosis.

■ Opt for live bio-yoghurt (or probiotic) yoghurt because it contains lactobacillus and bifida bacteria, which, if consumed regularly enough, can boost levels of 'friendly' probiotic bacteria in your bowel or colon. These promote efficient digestion and absorption of food, inhibit the growth of harmful bacteria (such as salmonella and E-coli, which can cause food poisoning) and help to combat the negative effects of stress, alcohol, highly processed foods and the imbalance that can be caused in the body by drugs such as antibiotics.

When it's good:

Any time, but a pot (or two) of yoghurt is particularly good after intense workouts as it's protein–carbohydrate combination encourages faster glycogen replenishment than carbohydrate alone.

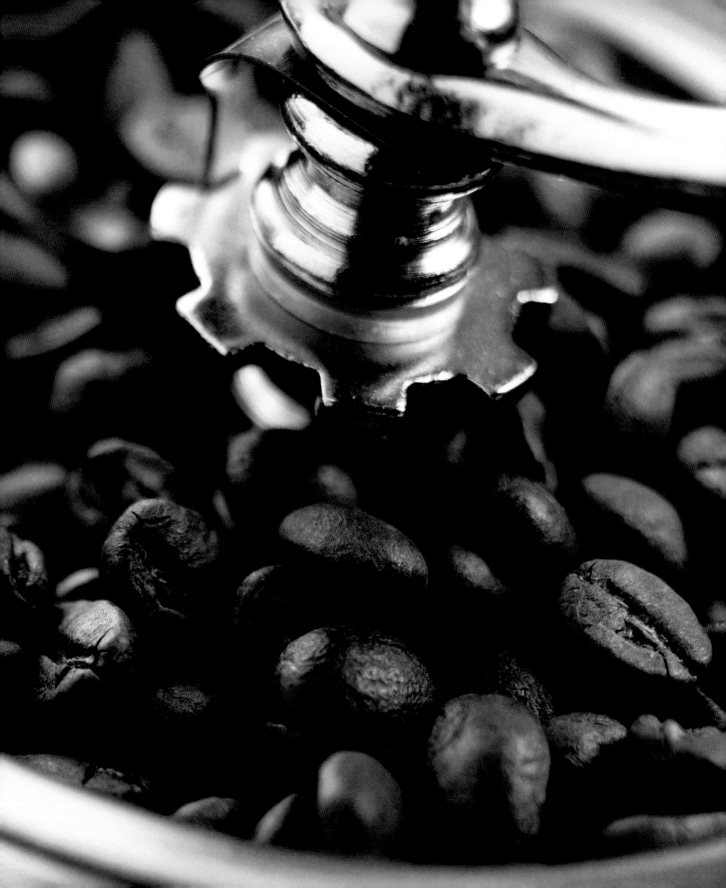

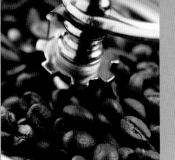

8 sports supplements

The vast array of supplements, all promising to benefit your health, physical performance or mental power, presents a confusing choice for regular exercisers. Many are advertised in fitness publications alongside impressive testimonials or sports celebrity endorsements, which can make the product's claims appear very convincing. But, despite the hype, many have little, if any, scientific backing. In this chapter you'll find an independent evaluation of the most popular supplements marketed to regular exercisers. Do they work? Do they live up to their claims? And are they safe?

Are supplements safe?

The problem with dietary supplements is that they are classified as foods so they don't have to undergo safety tests. Unlike medicines, there's no systematic regulation of supplements or herbal remedies, so there's no guarantee that a supplement lives up to its claims. Tests have found that some do not even contain the ingredients declared on the label; others may be contaminated with prohibited stimulants or substances. An IOC-funded 2001 survey of 634 supplements found 15 per cent were contaminated with banned substances, including steroids. UK Sport and the British Olympic Association caution athletes against taking any supplements.

WHICH PILLS ARE YOU POPPING?

The most popular supplements are multivitamins, according to surveys carried out by university researchers in the United States. The majority of regular exercisers take them, followed by carbohydrate/energy supplements, protein supplements, creatine and caffeine. Ephedrine, androstenedione, glutamine and HMB are also popular among strength athletes.

---

tip Evaluating a supplement

■ Don't be taken in by supplements that promise dramatic results. If the manufacturer's claims sound too good to be true, then they probably are.

■ Be sceptical of adverts that contain lots of technical jargon or unnecessary graphs. If the information isn't clear and factual, leave the supplement well alone.

■ Be wary of glossy adverts that rely on astonishing 'before' and 'after' photos rather than scientifically sound evidence for the supplement.

■ Ask the manufacturer for evidence and studies that support the supplement's claims. If the information isn't available, don't touch that supplement.

■ Check that any evidence is unbiased. Ideally, studies should have been carried out at a university, not funded solely by the manufacturer, and published in a reputable scientific journal.

■ Don't take a supplement that has been recommended only by word of mouth. Check out exactly what is in it and whether it works before you buy it. Ask an expert if you have any questions.

Antioxidant supplements

What's in them?

Antioxidant supplements contain various combinations of antioxidant nutrients and plant extracts, including beta-carotene, vitamin C, vitamin E, zinc, magnesium, copper, lycopene (pigment found in tomatoes), selenium, co-enzyme Q10, catechins (found in green tea), methionine (an amino acid) and anthocyanidins (pigments found in purple or red fruit).

What do they do?

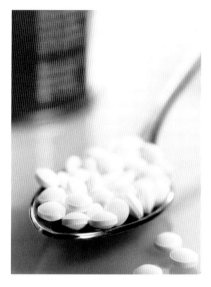

Antioxidants quench potentially harmful free radicals produced in the body. Although the body produces its own antioxidant enzymes, and levels increase with regular exercise, supplements may further boost these natural defences. Studies have linked a high intake of antioxidants from diet and supplements with a reduced risk of premature ageing, heart disease, certain cancers and cataracts. Supplements may help promote recovery after intense exercise and reduce post-exercise muscle soreness. Combinations of antioxidants are more effective than single antioxidant nutrients.

Do you need them?

A daily antioxidant supplement should not be a substitute for a healthy diet but it may give you increased protection from chronic diseases and speed your recovery after intense workouts. For best antioxidant protection, aim to eat at least five portions of fruit and vegetables daily – the more intense the colour, the higher the antioxidant content – as well as foods rich in essential fats (such as avocados, oily fish and pure vegetable oils) for their vitamin E content.

Are there any side effects?

Side effects are unlikely for antioxidant mixtures. Keep to the recommended dose on the label. When taking antioxidant supplements you should avoid vitamin C intakes over 1,000 mg due to the risk of stomach upsets, and selenium intakes over 900 micrograms due to the risk of toxicity.

Caffeine

What is it?

Caffeine is classed as a drug rather than a nutrient. However, it is often considered a nutritional supplement because it is found in many everyday foods and drinks such as coffee, black and green tea, cola, chocolate, certain energy and sports drinks and some energy gels. The caffeine content of coffee can vary enormously depending how you make it: a 2004 Food Standards Agency survey found that the caffeine content of brewed ground coffee ranged from 15–254 mg per cup.

HOW MUCH CAFFEINE?	
Drink/food source	Caffeine content mg per cup
Instant coffee	60 mg
Espresso	45–100 mg
Cafetière/filter coffee	60–120 mg
Tea	40 mg
Green tea	40 mg
Energy drinks	100 mg
Cola	40 mg
Energy gel	1 sachet: 25 mg
Dark chocolate	50 g bar: 40 mg
Milk chocolate	50 g bar: 12mg

What does it do?

Caffeine stimulates the release of the hormone adrenaline, which increases the levels of fatty acids in your bloodstream. During exercise, your muscles are able to use more fatty acids for fuel, which conserves valuable glycogen. This means you can work out longer without feeling tired. Caffeine is also a stimulant, boosting concentration, motivation and mental alertness, and masking fatigue. A University of Luton study showed that caffeine can improve endurance by an average of 12 per cent.

Do you need it?

Drinking the equivalent of two cups of coffee or a caffeinated energy drink about an hour before exercise may encourage the muscles to burn more fat and thus help you keep going for longer. Canadian researchers have found that taking more than two cups of coffee has no additional effect. Australian researchers have found that 1.5 milligrams of caffeine per kilogram – equivalent to 105 mg for a 70 kg (154 lb.) athlete – taken in divided doses (e.g. four caffeine-containing energy gels over two hours) throughout an intense workout, benefits performance in serious athletes.

To make the most of its benefits, drink coffee with no or only a small amount of (low-fat) milk because milk slows down its effects.

What are the side effects?

Side effects include anxiety, trembling and sleeplessness. Caffeine also increases your heart rate and breathing rate. Some people are more susceptible to the side effects than others. If you are sensitive to caffeine, it is best to avoid it.

Scientific research shows, on balance, no link between long-term caffeine use and health problems, such as hypertension and bone mineral loss. The connection between raised cholesterol levels and heavy coffee consumption is caused by certain fats in coffee, which are more pronounced in boiled coffee than instant or filter coffee.

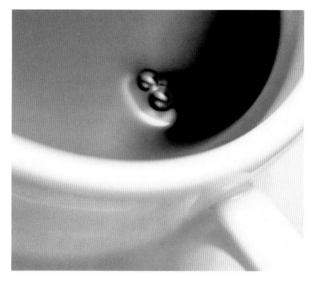

PRE-COMPETITION STRATEGY

If you're looking for that extra competitive edge, come off caffeine for a few days or significantly reduce your intake prior to a competition. This reduces your tolerance so that when you re-introduce caffeine to your system, you'll receive a greater response again. Just before the competition, take approximately 150–200 mg of caffeine from drinks, such as coffee (1–2 strong cups) or an energy/sports drink (1–2 cans). This may help you stay ahead of the pack or at least set a new PB.

Q&A

Question: *Does caffeine dehydrate you?*

Answer: Although caffeine is a diuretic, studies have shown that regular but moderate caffeine intake does not dehydrate the body as was once thought. Only if caffeine is taken in large doses – equivalent to more than three cups of coffee – or infrequently is it likely to have a noticeable diuretic effect. You can build up a tolerance to caffeine so its diuretic action becomes weakened if you consume it regularly.

Creatine

What's in it?

Creatine is a protein that is made naturally in the body from three amino acids (arginine, glycine and methionine) but is also found in meat and fish or taken in higher doses as a supplement. As a supplement, creatine is most commonly taken as a powder mixed with water, but liquid forms are also available.

What does it do?

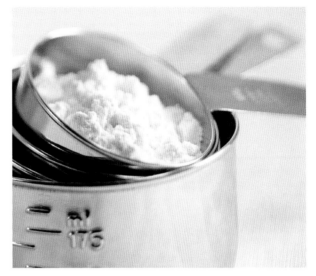

Creatine combines with phosphorus to form phosphocreatine (PC) in muscle cells. This is an energy-rich compound that fuels muscles during high-intensity activities, such as lifting weights or sprinting. Boosting PC levels with supplements enables you to sustain all-out effort longer than usual and recover faster between exertions or 'sets', resulting in greater strength and improved ability to do repeated sets. Studies have shown that creatine supplements can improve performance in high-intensity activities, as well as increase total and lean body weight.

Do you need it?

If you train with weights, sprint or do any sport that includes repeated sprints, jumps or throws (such as rugby and football), creatine supplements may help increase your strength, muscle mass and performance. But creatine doesn't work for everyone – several studies have found that creatine made no difference to performance, and it is unlikely to benefit endurance performance.

Are there any side effects?

The main side effect is weight gain. This is due partly to extra water in the muscle cells and partly to increased muscle tissue. While this is desirable for bodybuilders and people who work out with weights, it could be disadvantageous in sports where there is a critical ratio of body weight to speed (for example, for runners) or in weight-category sports. Some people suffer from water retention, particularly during the loading phase (see box on page 102). Other reported side effects include cramps and stomach discomfort, which may be due to dehydration rather than creatine. As larger-than-normal amounts of creatine need to be processed by the kidneys, there is a theoretical long-term risk of kidney damage. While short-term and low-dose creatine supplementation appears to be safe, the effects of long-term and/or high-dose creatine supplementation, alone or in combination with other supplements, remains unknown.

WHAT IS THE BEST WAY TO TAKE CREATINE?

While most manufacturers recommend loading up on creatine to boost levels in the muscles (20–25 g daily for 5 to 7 days), others suggest a more moderate dose over a longer period. Most of the early research on creatine used a loading dose of 20–25 g followed by a maintenance dose of 2–5 g daily. This method gives quick results but is more likely to produce side effects such as water retention. Also, the body has to work harder to process the excess creatine as less than 1 per cent of the dose ends up in the muscles; the remainder is excreted from the body. More recent research has shown that lower daily doses of 3–7 g, divided into four equal doses for 30 days, gives similar performance results but with less water retention. Canadian researchers found that 7 g daily produced significant increases in workout intensity, power output and muscle size over 21 days. On average, the volunteers gained 2.2 kg of lean body weight.

 Researchers recommend taking creatine with carbohydrate because the insulin spike produced by the carbohydrate drives more creatine into the muscles. The exact amount of carbohydrate is debatable but most studies have used between 30 and 90 g. Taking creatine supplements with meals is a cheaper and equally effective option to buying more expensive creatine-carbohydrate products.

Conjugated Linoleic Acid (CLA)

What's in it?

CLA is an unsaturated fatty acid, a mixture of linoleic acid (omega-6) isomers, found naturally in small amounts in full-fat milk, meat and cheese. Supplements are made from sunflower and safflower oils.

What does it do?

CLA may help reduce fat storage and increase fat burning. It is thought that CLA works by stimulating the enzyme hormone-sensitive lipase (which releases fat from fat cells) and suppressing the hormone lipoprotein lipase (which transports fat into fat cells). When combined with resistance training,

CLA may also increase muscle mass and strength. In the USA, University of Memphis researchers found that, compared with a placebo, CLA improved strength in experienced weight lifters. A study of novice bodybuilders at Kent State University in the USA found that six weeks of supplementation resulted in increased arm circumference, total muscle mass and overall strength compared with a placebo group.

Do you need it?

Taking 2–5 g per day may help reduce body fat and maintain or increase muscle mass.

Are there any side effects?

None have been reported to date.

Energy Bars

What are they?

Energy bars are essentially a concentrated from of carbohydrate, consisting mainly of maltodextrin, corn syrup, sugars, dried fruit or cereal. Most provide around 200 calories and 50 g of carbohydrate per bar with very little protein or fat.

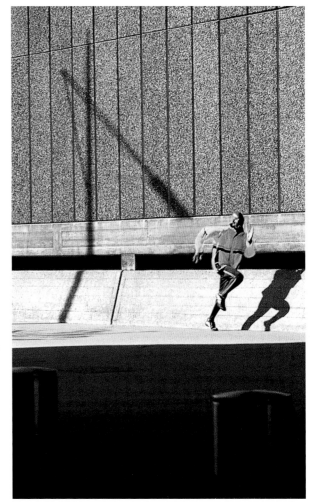

What do they do?

Energy bars provide a convenient energy fix, and solid carbohydrates are as good as liquid carbohydrates when it comes to fuelling before, during and after exercise. University of Sydney researchers found that low-glycaemic solid carbohydrates eaten before training improved endurance because they provide a sustained release of energy. Another Australian study with cyclists compared an energy bar (plus water) with a sports drink during exercise; it was found that both boosted blood sugar levels and endurance.

Researchers at Cornell University, New York, found that solid and liquid carbohydrates were, again, equally effective in promoting glycogen re-fuelling after intense and prolonged exercise.

Do you need them?

The main benefit of energy bars is their convenience: they are easy to carry for eating during or after exercise. Make sure that you have your bar with enough water (at least 250 ml) to replace fluids lost in sweat as well as to digest the bar. Check the label as some brands are loaded with high GI sugars (glucose or corn syrup), which produces a surge in blood sugar and insulin. The box below will help you choose the right bar.

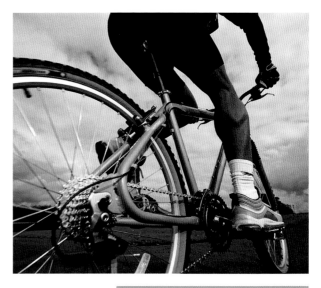

Are there any side effects?

There are no side effects except the risk of fat gain if you consume too many calories.

Energy gels

What are they?

Energy gels come in small squeezable sachets and have a 'gloopy' jelly-like texture. They consist almost entirely of simple sugars (such as fructose and glucose) and maltodextrin (a carbohydrate consisting of 4–20 glucose units). They may also contain sodium, potassium and, sometimes, caffeine. Most contain between 18 and 25 g of carbohydrate per sachet.

What do they do?

Gels provide a concentrated source of calories and carbohydrate and are designed to be consumed during endurance exercise. Studies show that consuming 30–60 g of carbohydrates per hour during prolonged exercise delays fatigue and improves endurance. This translates into 1–2 sachets per hour. One study showed that gels have a similar effect on blood sugar levels and performance as sports drinks.

HOW TO CHOOSE THE RIGHT ENERGY BAR

Choose a bar that contains between 30 and 60 g of carbohydrates.

Check that the bar contains no more than 5 g of fat per 200 calories. Fat slows digestion, which can make you feel heavy and nauseous during exercise.

Some of the bars are sticky and may adhere to your teeth. Make sure you rinse your mouth well with water after eating a bar. Better still; brush your teeth after a workout.

Energy bars are expensive. For a cheaper alternative, you may want to try cereal bars and breakfast bars (*see* pages 86–87).

Do you need them?

Gels are a convenient way of consuming carbohydrate during intense endurance exercise lasting longer than an hour. However, you need to drink around 350 ml of water with each 25 g of carbohydrate gel to dilute it to a 7 per cent carbohydrate solution in your stomach. Try half a gel with 175 ml – equivalent to about six big gulps – every 15 to 30 minutes. On the downside, some people dislike energy gels' texture, sweetness and intensity of flavour – it's really down to personal preference. You will also need to carry a bottle of water with you.

Are there any side effects?

Energy gels don't hydrate you so you must drink plenty of water with them. If you don't drink enough, you'll end up with a gelatinous gloop in your stomach. This drags water from your bloodstream into your stomach, increasing the risk of dehydration.

Fat burners, or thermogenics

What are they?

Fat-burning or 'diet' pills claim to speed your metabolism and shed body fat. The main ingredient is ephedrine, or ephedra (from the Chinese herb, ma huang). Ephedrine may also be found combined with caffeine and aspirin.

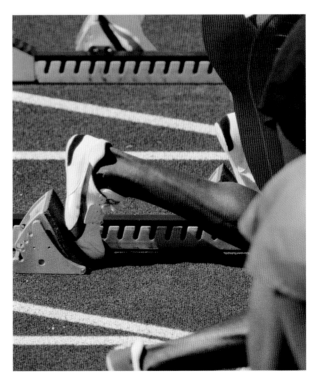

What do they do?

Ephedrine is chemically similar to amphetamines and is a powerful central nervous system stimulant. It makes you feel more alert and increases heart rate and blood pressure as well as speeding up metabolic rate and calorie burn. When ephedrine and caffeine are taken together they appear to boost each other's effects. Aspirin is also sometimes added as it may prolong the stimulant activity of the other two. No one knows the precise action but it is thought that when you take them, you temporarily supercharge the nervous system, causing an increase in heat production (or thermogenesis) and release of stored fat.

Studies have shown that these supplements do indeed enhance fat loss when taken with a low-calorie diet but this effect decreases over time. The problem is that they can also cause harmful side effects (see below).

Do you need them?

Ephedrine (or ma huang) is an addictive drug and I would strongly recommend avoiding any fat burner containing ephedrine because of the significant health risks. The International Olympic Committee (IOC) bans ephedrine. Exercise and good nutrition are the safest methods for burning fat.

Are there any side effects?

The doses necessary to cause a fat-burning effect are quite high and are associated with a number of risky side effects including an increased and irregular heart beat, a rise in blood pressure, irritability, dizziness and other symptoms of nervousness. More severe consequences such as heart attack, stroke and death have been reported in the medical press. Taking ephedrine with caffeine and aspirin further increases the chance of side effects.

Fat burners (ephedrine-free)

What are they?

Some fat-burning pills and capsules claim to mimic the effects of ephedrine, boost the metabolism and enhance fat loss, without harmful side effects. The most popular ingredients include citrus aurantium (synephrine or bitter orange extract), green tea extract and forskolin (a herb).

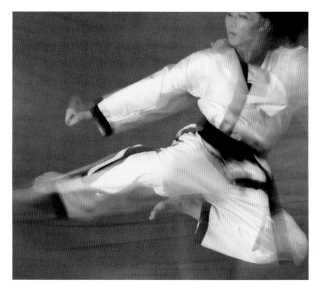

What do they do?

Citrus aurantium is related to ephedrine but has a much weaker stimulating effect on the nervous system. Green tea extract contains polyphenols (antioxidants) that may enhance fat burning and increase the metabolic rate. Initial research suggests that polyphenols may cause a greater proportion of fat (rather than carbohydrate) to be burned for energy. Forskolin extract also appears to boost metabolism and stimulate the release of stored fat.

Do you need them?

The research on ephedrine-free fat burners is only preliminary and any fat-burning boost they provide is relatively small. The doses used in some brands may be too small to provide a measurable effect. Again, sensible eating and exercise are likely to produce better weight loss results in the long term. Drinking green tea will boost your antioxidant intake but probably won't enhance fat burning.

Are there any side effects?

While the herbal alternatives to ephedrine are generally safer, you may get side effects with high doses. Citrus aurantium can increase blood pressure as much as, if not more than, ephedrine. High doses of forskolin may cause heart disturbances.

Glucosamine

What is it?

Glucosamine is found naturally in the body. It is an amino sugar involved in cartilage formation and repair. It is also one of the main substances in synovial fluid that lubricates and provides nutrients for joint structures. Glucosamine supplements are made from crab, lobster and shrimp shells.

What does it do?

As the body ages, cartilage loses its elasticity and cushioning properties for joints, which may result in stiffness, immobility and pain. Supplements may help repair damaged tendons, cartilage and soft tissue. Glucosamine stimulates the cartilage cells to produce proteoglycans (building blocks) that repair joint structures.

Do you need it?

Glucosamine supplements can help relieve stiffness, pain and improve mobility in people with joint problems, including osteoarthritis. The recommendation is to take 500 mg with food three times a day. It may take three to eight weeks to produce noticeable results. Glucosamine sulphate is sometimes combined with chrondroitin sulphate, which also helps stimulate cartilage repair mechanisms and inhibit enzymes that break down cartilage.

Are there any side effects?

May include stomach discomfort and intestinal gas.

Glutamine

What is it?

Glutamine is a non-essential amino acid found abundantly in the muscle cells and blood. Glutamine supplements can be taken as powders, which are mixed with water or added to a protein shake, and capsules.

What does it do?

Glutamine is needed for cell growth as well as serving as a fuel for the immune system. During periods of heavy training or stress, blood levels of glutamine fall, weakening the immune system and putting you at risk of infection. Muscle levels of glutamine also fall, which results in loss of muscle tissue, despite continued training.

Do you need it?

Manufacturers claim that glutamine has a protein-sparing effect during intense training. But the evidence for glutamine is divided. Some studies have shown that taking supplements of glutamine immediately after heavy training or an exhaustive event (such as a marathon) can help you recover faster, reduce muscle soreness and cut your risk of catching colds and other infections. Other studies have failed to show any benefits; for example, Canadian researchers found glutamine produced no increase in strength or muscle mass compared with a placebo.

Are there any side effects?

No side effects have currently been identified.

HMB (beta-hydroxy beta-methyl butyrate)

What is it?

HMB is the by-product of the body's normal breakdown of leucine, an essential amino acid.

What does it do?

HMB is involved with the repair and growth of muscle cells. Studies in the 1990s at Iowa State University in the USA suggested that HMB may reduce muscle breakdown and damage, promote faster muscle repair and increase muscle mass. But these benefits have not been found in all athletes, particularly more experienced athletes. One Australian study found that six weeks of HMB supplementation had no effect on the strength or muscle mass gains of well-conditioned athletes.

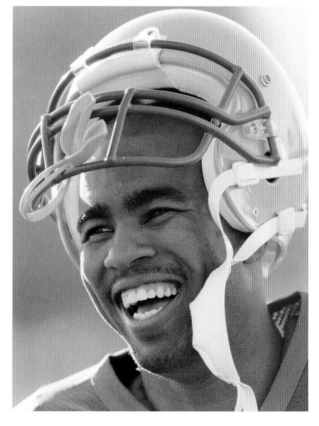

Do you need it?

If you're new to lifting weights, HMB may help boost your strength and build muscle. But it is unlikely to be useful to more experienced gym goers.

Are there any side effects?

No side effects have yet been found.

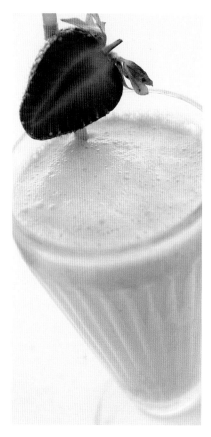

Meal replacement shakes

What's in them?

Meal replacement shakes contain a mixture of milk proteins (usually whey protein and/or casein), carbohydrate (maltodextrin and/or sugars), vitamins and minerals. Some brands also contain small amounts of oil and other nutrients that claim to boost performance.

What do they do?

They provide a well-balanced and convenient alternative to solid food.

Do you need them?

Meal replacement shakes will not necessarily improve your performance but they can be a helpful and convenient addition (rather than replacement) to your diet if you struggle to eat enough real food, you need to eat on the move or you need the extra nutrients they provide.

Are there any side effects?

Side effects are unlikely.

Multivitamin and mineral supplements

What's in them?

Multivitamin and mineral pills contain a mixture of micronutrients. In food-state supplements, the micronutrients are combined with a yeast base to mimic the form the nutrient takes in food and increase amounts absorbed by the body.

What do they do?

They will make up any nutritional shortfall in your diet and boost your nutritional status. If your diet is poor, supplements will help improve health, resistance to infection and post-workout recovery. However, there is no evidence that high doses enhance exercise performance.

Do you need them?

Many people would probably benefit from taking a supplement, but popping a pill can't erase the health effects of a poor diet and sedentary lifestyle. Go for real food first and take regular exercise. If you workout intensely several times a week, your requirements for many vitamins and minerals will be greater than the recommended daily allowance (RDA) so supplements may help meet your needs better. A deficiency of any vitamin and mineral will impair your health as well as your performance.

Are there any side effects?

Taking vitamin and mineral supplements is generally harmless but the Food Standards Agency does publish guidelines on safe upper levels. These include a warning not to exceed 10 mg per day of chromium picolinate. Other possible side effects of exceeding recommended daily amounts include:

- taking more than 1,000 mg of vitamin C daily may cause an upset stomach
- taking more than 17 mg of iron daily may cause constipation
- taking more than 10 mg of vitamin B6 over a long period may lead to numbness and persistent pins and needles
- high doses of vitamin A should be avoided during pregnancy as this may result in birth defects
- vitamin D in high doses may cause high blood pressure.

As a general rule, never take more than 10 times the RDA of vitamins A and D, and no more than the RDA

for any mineral. Check the quantities on the label and do not exceed the upper safe levels shown in the Essential Guide to Vitamins and Minerals (pages 19–21).

Prohormones/steroid precursors

What are they?

Prohormone supplements, including DHEA, androstenedione (or andro for short) and norandrostenedione are marketed to bodybuilders and other athletes looking to increase strength and muscle mass.

What do they do?

Manufacturers claim the supplements will increase testosterone levels in the body and produce similar muscle-building effects to anabolic steroids, but without the side effects.

However, researchers at Iowa State University in the USA found that andro and DHEA supplements do not elevate testosterone, nor do they live up to their claims of increasing strength and muscle mass. Higher doses than those recommended on supplement labels may raise testosterone but there is no evidence that this results in greater muscle mass or strength.

Do you need them?

It is unlikely that prohormones work and they may produce unwanted side effects (see opposite). Furthermore, their contents cannot always be guaranteed: in tests carried out by the International Olympic Committee laboratory in Cologne, Germany, it was found that 15 per cent of supplements contained substances that would lead to a failed drugs test, including nandrolone, despite them not being listed on the label.

Are there any side effects?

Studies have found that most prohormones increase oestrogen (which can lead to breast development) and decrease HDL (good cholesterol) levels. Some supplements include anti-oestrogen substances such as chrysin but there is, as yet, no evidence that they work.

Protein supplements

What's in them?

Protein supplements can be divided into three main categories: protein powders (which are mixed with milk or water into a shake), ready-to-drink shakes and high-protein bars. They may contain whey protein, casein, soy protein or a mixture of these.

What do they do?

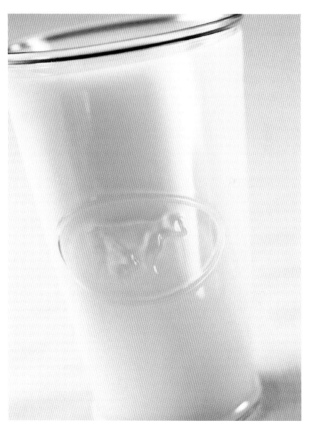

Protein supplements provide a concentrated source of protein to supplement usual food intake. Whey protein is derived from milk and contains high levels of the essential amino acids (*see* page 11), which are readily digested, absorbed and retained by the body for muscle repair. Whey protein may also help enhance the immune function. Casein, also derived from milk, provides a slower-digested protein, as well as high levels of amino acids. It may help protect against muscle breakdown during intense training.

Do you need them?

Protein supplements can help make up any protein shortfall in the diet of regular exercisers who have higher protein needs than normal, such as strength and power athletes or vegetarian athletes. Experts recommend a protein intake of between 1.4 and 1.8 g per kilogram of bodyweight per day, equivalent to 98–126 g daily for a 70 kg person.

Most regular exercisers can get enough protein from between two and four daily portions of chicken, fish, dairy products, eggs and pulses (*see* chapter 1, pages 1–26). Vegetarians can meet their protein needs by eating a variety of plant proteins (tofu, quorn, beans, lentils, nuts) each day. (*See* box on page 11 for the protein content of various foods.) Use protein supplements if you are unable to meet your protein needs from food alone.

Are there any side effects?

An excessive intake of protein, whether from food or supplements, is not harmful but offers no health or performance advantage. Concerns about excess protein harming the liver and kidneys or causing calcium loss from the bones have been disproved.

Sports drinks

What are they?

Sports drinks fall into two categories:

- fluid replacement drinks containing up to 8 g of carbohydrate per 100 ml.
- energy drinks containing 12–20 g of carbohydrate per 100 ml.

Both categories provide water, carbohydrate (in the form of sucrose, glucose, fructose and maltodextrin) and electrolytes (sodium and potassium). They are designed to replace body fluids more rapidly than plain water.

What do they do?

The sugars and maltodextrin (complex carbohydrates derived from cornstarch, consisting of 8–20 glucose units per molecule) in sports drinks help speed the absorption of water from the gut into the bloodstream. The carbohydrate concentration may be either **isotonic** (the same concentration as body fluids) or **hypotonic** (more dilute than body fluids). The purpose of sodium in sports drinks is to stimulate drinking (salt makes you thirsty) and help the body better retain the fluid. Research carried out by the University of Texas found that drinking water during one hour of cycling improved performance by 6 per cent compared with no water, but drinking a sugar-containing drink resulted in a 12 per cent improvement on performance.

tip **How to choose the right protein bar**
- For best refuelling, go for a bar that contains between two to three times as much carbohydrate as protein.
- Check the bar contains whey protein, casein or soy protein, rather than hydrolysed gelatine (which is made from the hooves of cows and horses!).
- Steer clear of bars that list corn syrup, sugar syrup, glucose or sweeteners as their main ingredients.
- Check that the bar contains no more than 5 g of fat per 200 calories and doesn't include palm kernel oil or hydrogenated fat.

Do you need them?

- If you are working out continually for longer than 60 minutes, a sports drink instead of water may help you keep going longer or work harder. Drink between 0.5–1.0 litres per hour.

- If you haven't eaten for more than four hours, try a pre-workout sports drink.

- If you are training for between 1 and 2 hours, choose fluid replacement drinks containing less than 8 g of sugar per 100 ml.

- For intense workouts lasting longer than two hours, choose an energy drink based on maltodextrin.

- For a less expensive alternative, try mixing fruit juice with equal quantities of water. This produces an isotonic drink with around 6 g of sugar per 100 ml. Add a pinch (one-quarter of a teaspoon) of ordinary salt if you sweat heavily.

Are there any side effects?
Side effects are unlikely, provided you stick to the recommended dilution on the label. Avoid caffeine- and ephedrine-containing drinks if you are sensitive to their side effects.

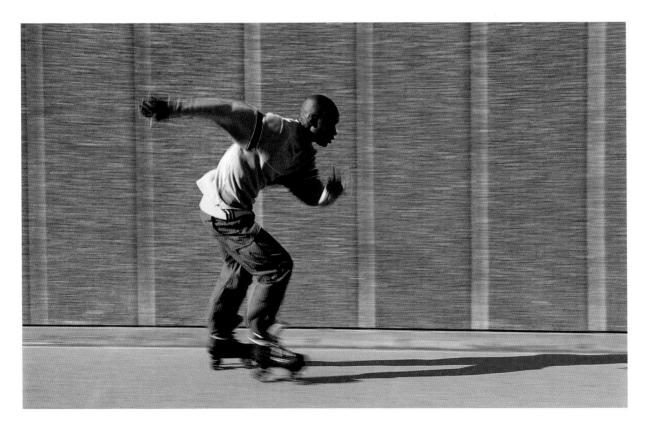

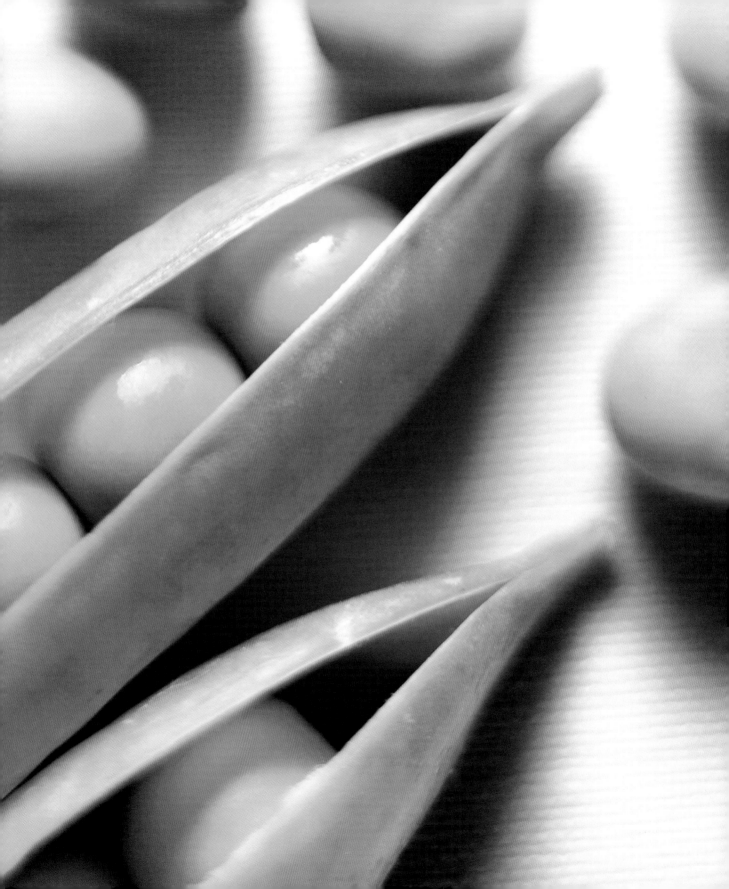

9 nutrition strategy for competitions

What you eat and drink in the weeks and days before a competition makes a big difference to your performance. Start your nutritional strategy as early in your preparations as possible – this will help you train smarter – then fine-tune your diet in the last week before the event. Rehearse in training what you plan to eat and drink on the day of the event and never try anything new. Research the foods and drinks to be provided at the venue so you can test them out beforehand. Alternatively, take your own supplies. Read on for lots of tried and tested tips for pre-competition nutrition.

Travelling nutrition

For most competitors, big events require a great deal of travelling. You can spend hours in a car, on a motorway, in a tailback on a hot day – in short, it can be a psychological nightmare. It can also negatively affect your glycogen stores and hydration if you don't prepare a travelling nutrition strategy, and this requires a certain degree of organisation.

Don't rely on finding the right foods at outlets en route or at the venue – healthy choices are often limited at these places. It is best to take your own supplies for the journey as well as for race day. Snacks for eating on the move include:

- sandwiches filled with chicken, tuna or cheese with salad
- banana and peanut butter sandwiches
- rice cakes, oatcakes and wholemeal crackers
- bottles of water
- cartons of fruit juice
- yoghurt drinks
- individual cheese portions
- small bags of nuts (peanuts, cashews, almonds)
- fresh fruit (apples, bananas, grapes)
- mini-boxes of raisins

tip

Coping with pre-competition nerves

Most athletes get pre-competition nerves, which can reduce the appetite and result in problems such as nausea, diarrhoea and stomach cramps. If you find it difficult to eat solid food during this time, try the following:

- *liquid meals such as flavoured milk, meal replacement products (protein-carbohydrate drinks), sports drinks, milk shakes, yoghurt drinks and fruit smoothies*
- *smooth, semi-liquid foods such as puréed fruit (e.g. apple purée, mashed banana, apple and apricot purée), yoghurt, porridge, custard and rice pudding*
- *bland foods such as semolina, mashed potato or porridge made from cornmeal or ground rice.*

- a fruit bar or liquorice bar

- sesame snaps

- prepared vegetable crudités (carrots, peppers, cucumber, celery).

If you're travelling abroad, take care to avoid common food poisoning culprits (chicken, seafood and meat dishes) unless you're sure they have been properly cooked and heated to a high temperature. At all costs, avoid anything lukewarm. You should also peel fruit and vegetables, stick to bottled water and avoid ice in drinks.

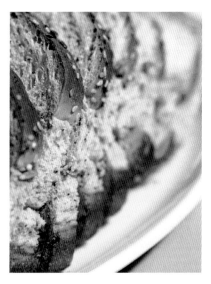

SUITABLE RESTAURANT MEALS AND FAST FOODS WHEN TRAVELLING TO AN EVENT

- Simple pasta dishes with tomato sauce

- Rice and stir-fried vegetable dishes

- Pizza with simple tomato and vegetable toppings

- Simple noodle dishes

- Jacket potatoes with cheese

- Pancakes with syrup

RESTAURANT MEALS AND FAST FOODS TO AVOID

- Burgers and chips

- Chicken nuggets

- Pasta with creamy or oily sauces

- Takeaway curries

- Takeaway kebabs

- Battered fish and chips

- Lukewarm chicken, turkey, meat, fish or seafood dishes

- Hot dogs

- Fried chicken meals

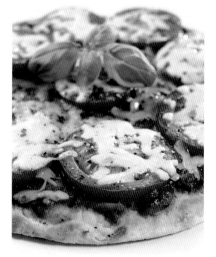

Running events

The week before the race

Your aim during the week before a race is to fill your muscles with the glycogen they'll need for the race. Starting the race with high glycogen levels will help you to keep going longer before you get tired.

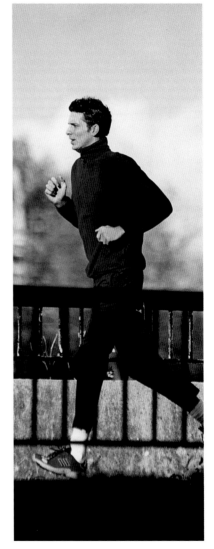

---

tip   **Race preparation: the week before**

- *Taper your training.* For the last few days before the race, reduce your mileage and drop your training intensity. Rest completely for the day or two before the race.
- *Downsize your meals.* You'll be training less as the week progresses, so you may need to drop your calorie intake a little. Do this by cutting out foods containing saturated fats and 'empty calories', such as confectionery, pastries, crisps and fast foods.
- *Carb up.* Change the nutrient mix of your pre-race diet so you get more of your calories from carbohydrate (60–70 per cent) and fewer from fat (less than 15–20 per cent), the balance coming from protein. Remember, it's the proportion of carbohydrates not the total calories that needs to go up.
- *Eat little and often.* Small, frequent meals will be easier to digest and will prevent you feeling bloated. Avoid big meals and don't eat too much of any one food.
- *Slow burn.* Choose low-glycaemic meals and foods that will promote better glycogen storage. Carbohydrates eaten with some protein or healthy fat (such as potatoes with chicken, pasta with fish, rice with tofu) give a longer, slower energy release compared with carbohydrates on their own.
- *Get bottle savvy.* Keep well hydrated by drinking at least 2 litres of water per day.

The day before the race

By now, your muscle glycogen stores should be almost fully stocked and you should be feeling rested. Your goals for the day before the race are to top-up your glycogen stores, stay well-hydrated and avoid any pitfalls that may jeopardise your performance the next day.

CARBOHYDRATE LOADING

Carbohydrate loading – increasing glycogen stores above normal – may improve performance during races lasting 90 minutes or longer. However, it won't help you run faster in shorter runs. In fact, the heaviness associated with elevated glycogen stores may hinder your performance. You can try carbohydrate loading during the days before a big event. Rehearse in training several weeks beforehand.

In the first three days, eat a normal diet.

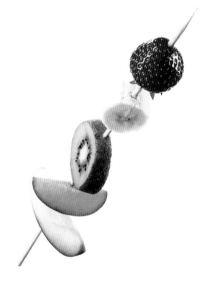

- On the second day, run at a hard pace for 90 minutes. This will deplete your muscle glycogen stores.

- On the third and fourth days, run for 45 minutes at the same intensity. This will further deplete your muscle glycogen.

- On the fifth and sixth days, run only very short distances.

- On the day before the race, rest.

- During the three days before the event, eat a high carbohydrate diet providing 7–10 g of carbohydrate per day. This will fill your muscle glycogen stores.

tip

Race preparation: the day before

- *Graze. Eat little and often throughout the day. Choose high-carbohydrate, low-fat, moderate-protein meals to avoid overburdening your digestive system.*

- *Avoid feasting. It's not a good idea to over-indulge the night before a race as this can play havoc with your digestive system and keep you awake at night. You may also feel sluggish the next day.*

- *Stick with familiar foods. Eat only foods that you know agree with you and eat them in normal-sized amounts. Don't try anything new.*

- *Avoid alcohol. Alcohol is a diuretic and, if you over-indulge, you may feel below par the next day.*

- *Beware of the gas. Avoid gas-forming foods (or combinations of food) such as baked beans and other pulses, cruciferous vegetables (broccoli, Brussels sprouts, cauliflower), bran cereals and spicy foods the night before the race. They may make you feel uncomfortable.*

- *Take to the bottle. Keep a water bottle handy so you remember to drink regularly throughout the day. This is especially important if you are travelling to the race venue on this day, as it is easy to forget to drink.*

On race day

By now, your muscle glycogen stores should be fully stocked and you should feel ready to go! All that remains to be done before the race is to top-up your liver glycogen stores at breakfast time (liver glycogen is normally depleted during the overnight fast), replace any fluids lost overnight and keep your blood sugar level steady.

> **tip**
>
> ### Race preparation: the day of the race
>
> - *Eat early. It takes 3–4 hours for food to digest so schedule your pre-race meal early. If your race starts at 9 am, have breakfast at 6 am.*
> - *Eat light. Aim for 25–50 g of carbohydrate for each hour before the start of the race, depending on your body weight and the race duration (see box right for suggestions). Carbohydrate-rich foods, such as porridge, cereal, toast and fruit, are good choices. Include a little protein or healthy fat to reduce the glycaemic response and give a slow, steady energy release. If you can't eat because of pre-race nerves, have an extra bedtime snack the night before or try a liquid meal (for example, a meal replacement shake, milkshake, smoothie or yoghurt drink) for breakfast, which will empty from your stomach faster than solid food.*
> - *Drink before you race. Drink at least 500 ml of water, a sports drink or diluted fruit juice (1 part juice to 1–2 parts water) during the two hours before the race, then another 125–250 ml just before the race.*

PRE-RACE MEALS

Eat the following with 150–300 ml of water or diluted fruit juice (1 part juice to 1–2 parts water).

- Porridge with raisins and honey
- Cereal with milk and bananas
- Toast with jam and a milky drink
- Pancakes or waffles with honey
- Meal replacement shake
- Meal replacement bar
- Protein shake and fresh fruit
- Yoghurt and fresh fruit
- Fruit smoothie
- Yoghurt drink

During the race

Drink every 20 minutes

For races lasting more than 30 minutes, begin drinking within the first 30 minutes instead of trying to rehydrate later. As a rough guide, aim to drink 125–250 ml – equivalent to about six gulps – every 15 to 20 minutes or according to thirst. Use whichever drinking method you have trained with. Be extra diligent in hot and humid weather.

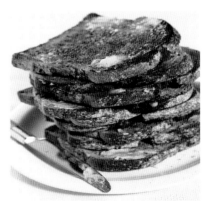

Slow down through the fluid stations

Walk or slow down to drink at least a cupful at every fluid station – more in hot weather. If you try to run you will end up spilling most of the drink. Squeezing the cup into a funnel makes it easier to drink. Don't be tempted to miss out the early fluid stations to gain valuable time – dehydration later on will slow you down even more.

Choose the right drink

If there is choice, select plain water for races lasting less than an hour and sports drinks for longer events. Stick with whatever you have used in training and don't try anything new.

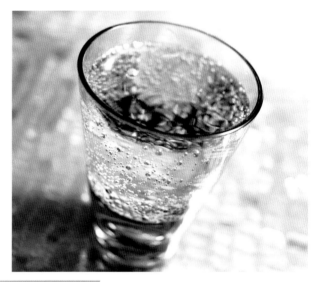

Q&A

Question: *Is it possible to drink too much water?*

Answer: During long endurance events such as marathons, over-hydrating yourself by constantly drinking water may dilute the blood so that sodium levels fall, a condition known as hyponatraemia. Although this is quite rare the condition is potentially fatal. The national governing body for track and field in the United States, USA Track and Field, cautions against drinking huge amounts of water in events lasting more than four hours; they advise that runners should be guided by their thirst and drink sports drinks with sodium. For most runners, however, there is a greater risk of dehydration than of over-hydration.

Q&A

Question: *I've noticed a lot of runners pouring water over their head. Would this stop me becoming dehydrated?*

Answer: Pouring water or squeezing a sponge over your head will help to cool you down but it won't help keep you hydrated. Drinking fluids will replenish sweat losses and regulate body temperature more effectively than pouring it over your skin. Do both if you want, but if you have to make a choice it is better to gulp a drink.

After the race

Congratulations! You have made it past the finishing line. However, your nutrition strategy isn't over yet; you still have to replenish your fluid losses and depleted glycogen stores. This is especially important if you plan to be active the next day and want to move around without difficulty tomorrow.

Drink, drink and drink

Start with water or, if you have been running for longer than 60 minutes, a sports (carbohydrate) drink. You need to replace the fluid you have lost but you won't know exactly how much without a set of scales. For every 0.5 kg of bodyweight lost you need to drink 750 ml of fluid. Try to drink around 500 ml, little and often, in the first 30 minutes after the race, and then keep gulping every 5 to 10 minutes until you are passing fairly clear urine again. You should be able to pass urine within two hours of a race. If you pass only a small volume of dark yellow urine, or if you are headachy and nauseous, then you need to keep drinking. If you are dehydrated, sports drinks or diluted fruit juice (with a pinch of salt added) are the best option.

Grab a snack

Choose a high-carbohydrate snack and aim to consume 1 g of carbohydrate per kilogram of bodyweight – equivalent to 70 g for a 70 kg runner – within the first 30 minutes. It does not matter whether the carbohydrate is in solid or liquid form – have whatever feels right (see box right for suggestions). Including a little protein with the carbohydrate will speed glycogen recovery.

Keep eating

Continue eating a similar-sized snack every two hours until your proper meal. This will promote faster recovery. It takes at least 24 hours to replenish glycogen stores after a short run but up to seven days after a marathon.

Don't overeat!

Even if you feel ravenous, choose your post-race meal wisely. Fried and fatty food could hinder your recovery and make you feel bloated. Stick to easily digested meals, such as pasta with tomato sauce, jacket potatoes with tuna or cottage cheese, chicken sandwiches or stir-fries.

POST-RACE SNACKS

Eat the following with 150–300 ml of water or diluted fruit juice (1 part juice to 1–2 parts water):

- Cereal bar or sports bar
- Fruit loaf (see recipe on page 192)
- Fruit bar
- Meal replacement shake
- Yoghurt drink
- Fresh fruit
- Dried fruit and nuts
- Chocolate-coated raisins or nuts
- Jam sandwich, roll or bagel

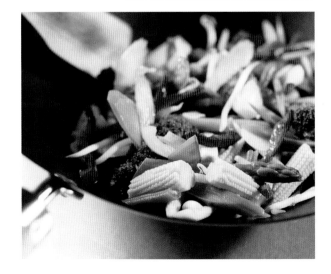

Q&A

Question: *How can I avoid 'hitting the wall' during a marathon?*

Answer: 'Hitting the wall' occurs when the muscles run out of glycogen and blood sugar levels fall below normal. At this stage you are in real trouble. The body needs carbohydrate to burn fat, and when there are no carbohydrates the brain and nervous system can't work properly. This makes exercise difficult if not impossible. You may feel weak, dizzy, nauseous and disorientated.

Here's how to avoid hitting the wall. Consume carbohydrate at regular intervals during your run, aiming to have 30–60 g of carbohydrate for every hour of exercise. This is equivalent to drinking 500–1,000 ml of sports drink (containing 60 g of carbohydrate per litre) each hour. Take regular sips and start drinking early as it takes about 30 minutes for the carbohydrate to reach your active muscles. This will help to keep your blood sugar levels steady and fuel your active muscles during that last stage of the race.

Question: *I have no appetite after a run and I certainly don't feel like eating. Should I wait until I'm hungry or force myself to eat?*

Answer: A lot of runners find they have little appetite after racing. Running (along with other types of intense exercise) elevates body temperature and diverts blood away from the digestive system, which in turn depresses the appetite. If you want to recover faster, you should consume some carbohydrate within the first 30 minutes after a race or, at the very least, within two hours. Try a liquid meal, such as a meal replacement shake, milkshake, smoothie or yoghurt drink. You'll feel better for it the next day.

Question: *I sometimes suffer from diarrhoea on long runs. What causes it and how can I prevent it?*

Answer: The 'trots' or 'runs' is common among endurance runners. Studies have shown that as many as one in four marathon runners experience it. The most likely explanation is that the lower gut (colon) becomes starved of oxygen during a long run due to a reduced blood flow. Blood is diverted away from the gut to the muscles and the skin, where more blood is required. This can result in spasmodic contractions of the colon. Being dehydrated will make the situation worse as the reduced blood volume means that even less blood is available to the gut.

The best strategy to prevent diarrhoea is to drink plenty of water before and during a run. Make sure that you drink during the early stages. It is also a good idea to avoid eating high-fibre foods, especially bran and wholegrain cereals, pulses and dried fruit, too close to the time of your run. These may loosen the stools and trigger bowel movements, a situation made worse by pre-race nerves. Caffeine and sorbitol sometimes have a laxative effect so you may also wish to avoid drinks and foods containing them. Keeping a food and training diary can help you work out which foods you can tolerate and which you need to avoid before a run.

Q&A

Question: *I often get cramps in my calves during a run. Is there anything I can eat or drink to stop this happening?*

Answer: Muscle cramps may be caused by several factors, including dehydration, increased body temperature and electrolyte (sodium/potassium) imbalance. Drink plenty of fluids before and during a run to offset dehydration. Sports drinks that contain sodium and potassium may help prevent cramps; alternatively, try diluted fruit juice with a pinch of ordinary salt.

Question: *Despite doing a lot of running, I have cellulite. Is it different from ordinary fat and is there a special diet I could follow to help get rid of it?*

Answer: You might be reassured to learn that cellulite affects 85 per cent of women and over 95 per cent of women aged over 30 years. Even exercise fanatics can be plagued by it. Cellulite is simply fat. The reason it appears dimpled and puckered is that it lies very close to the skin's surface and is criss-crossed by weak collagen strands that aren't very effective at supporting fat cells. This results in the characteristic bulging appearance of cellulite. The reason women get cellulite far more than men is the female hormone oestrogen, which favours fat storage on the thighs and bottom; hence women tend to put weight on in these areas. Inactivity, loss of muscle tone and excess calories are major contributors to the formation of cellulite. A healthy but careful calorie consumption combined with cardiovascular and resistence exercise is the only proven way to beat cellulite. There is no evidence that it is caused by 'toxins' or that following a detox diet reduces cellulite. However, cutting back on processed foods or those high in sugar, salt and fat will help reduce cellulite.

Cycling events

The week before the race

What you eat and drink during the week before a race can make a big difference to your performance. You goals are to maximise your muscle glycogen stores and keep yourself well hydrated.

Train less

Taper your training gradually. For the last few days of the week before a race, you should be cutting time in the saddle by half and then resting completely for the last day or two. If you don't reduce your training, you risk using

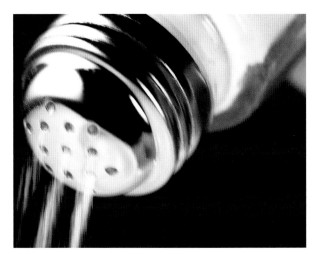

the carbohydrate you're eating to fuel your training rides instead of stockpiling it for the big event.

Carb up

Increase the amount of carbohydrate in your diet and reduce fat calories in a corresponding amount. Tipping the balance a little more in favour of carbohydrates (roughly 60–70 per cent carbohydrate calories) will boost glycogen levels and give you more fuel for the event. Tapering training along with increasing carbohydrate intake can increase your endurance by as much as 20 per cent.

Drink plenty

Make sure that you drink at least 2 litres per day. Dehydration is cumulative, so if you fail to drink sufficient amounts during the days leading up to a race, you could be dehydrated on the day of the race.

Avoid big meals

Eating too much in one meal will reduce the amount of glycogen stored and increase the chances of fat gain. Try to stick to regular meal times during the final week, to avoid stomach upsets.

Learn to eat and drink in the saddle

If you don't already, you will need to practise drinking from a water bottle or eating snacks while riding. Work out how to keep your balance without swerving while you drink or eat with one hand. Most cyclists move one hand to the centre of the handlebars (*see* box opposite).

The day before the race

The day before the race is your final chance to top-up muscle glycogen stores. It is also important to stay hydrated and avoid eating or drinking anything that may jeopardise your performance.

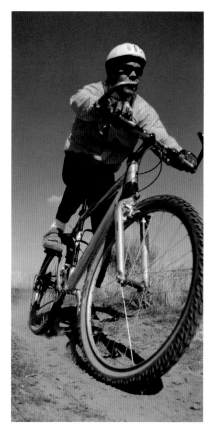

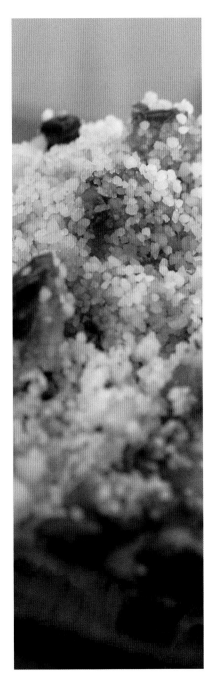

tip

How to eat and drink in the saddle

■ *Practise riding without holding on to the handlebars so that you can balance more easily while you eat and drink.*

■ *On long rides, wearing a specially designed pack that contains a plastic bladder (such as a camel pack) will enable you to drink without having to take your hands off the handlebars. You can also carry larger volumes of drink in a camel pack without needing to stop off to refill your bottle.*

■ *In hot weather, add ice cubes to your drink or freeze half the bottle (or camel pack) overnight and top it up before you get on your bike.*

■ *You can carry small snacks in the pockets of your jersey.*

■ *You can open food bars and undo packets before you set off; this will enable you to get at the food easily with one hand during the ride.*

■ *Peel fruit and wrap in foil for easy access.*

■ *Wrap dried fruit and biscuits in foil or small re-sealable plastic bags.*

■ *Soft-textured bars may be wrapped around the handlebars for easy access.*

tip

Race preparation: the day before

■ *Eat small. Divide your food into smaller, more frequent meals. Grazing will maximise glycogen storage without making you feel bloated and heavy.*

■ *Don't try new foods. The last thing you want before a race is a stomach upset so stick to familiar foods. Choose fairly plain foods, such as fish and rice or baked potato with cottage cheese, and avoid spicy and salty foods such as crisps, takeaways, ready-made sauces and ready-meals.*

■ *Keep drinking. Drink plenty of fluid throughout the day. Your urine should be pale or almost clear.*

■ *Avoid gas! Steer clear of gas-forming foods, such as baked beans, lentils and other pulses, cauliflower, Brussels sprouts, bran cereals and spicy foods. Eating them could give you an uncomfortable ride the next day.*

■ *Don't party. Be careful not to over-indulge the evening before your race. A large meal – even if high in carbohydrate – could make you feel sluggish the next day. If you must drink alcohol, restrict yourself to a maximum of 2 units, otherwise you risk dehydration and a hangover on race day. Better still, avoid alcohol altogether.*

On race day

On the day of the race, your muscle glycogen levels should be fully stocked and you should be feeling full of energy. However, what you eat just before the race is crucial. Consuming carbohydrate, particularly before longer races, provides energy for hard-working muscles. Carbohydrate will replenish the store of glycogen in the liver and keep blood sugar levels up.

Eat a good breakfast

Eat your pre-race meal two to four hours before the start of the race otherwise you may suffer stomach cramps during the race. This is because your digestive system has a reduced blood flow during the race, which makes it very difficult to digest large meals. Eat a moderate-sized carbohydrate-based breakfast that is also low in fat and contains some protein. Aim for 150–200 g of carbohydrate before a long ride; for short rides under two hours, you may need only 75–150 g. If you find it difficult to eat solid food when you're feeling nervous, try a liquid meal instead (*see* box on 'Pre-race meals' right). Skipping the pre-race meal may leave you low in energy during the final stages of the race.

Go easy on the fibre!

Steer clear of bran and high-fibre cereals, especially if you are feeling nervous. Cereal fibre may loosen the stools and cause more bowel movements than normal.

Drink

Make sure that you are properly hydrated by drinking 400–600 ml of water, a sports drink or diluted fruit juice (1 part juice to 1–2 parts water) during the two hours before the race. Your urine should be a very pale yellow by the start time. It is also wise to top-up with a further cupful of fluids just before you set off.

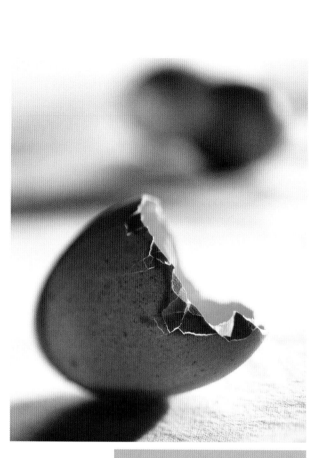

PRE-RACE MEALS

- Cereal with dried fruit and milk
- Scrambled egg on toast
- Porridge with fruit
- Toasted bagels or muffins and a milky drink
- Meal replacement shake with fruit
- Homemade milkshake
- Smoothie made with fruit and yoghurt

During the race

Drink every 15 to 20 minutes

Start drinking early in the race, ideally in the first 15 to 20 minutes. Your goal is to continue drinking little and often, aiming for 150–350 ml every 15 to 20 minutes. Remember, wind-chill and rapid evaporation of sweat can mask feelings of dehydration. Don't wait until you feel thirsty, as this is a poor indicator of your fluid needs.

Drink only what you know

Drink whatever you are used to drinking in training. As a rule of thumb, water is fine for rides lasting 60 to 90 minutes; sports drinks are better for longer races. However, do not try anything different – even if it is freely provided by the race organisers – in case it doesn't agree with you under race conditions.

Fuel in the saddle

For rides lasting longer than 90 minutes, you will need food or a sports drink to keep your blood sugar levels up. Try to consume 750–1,000 ml an hour. Alternatively, eat energy gels, bars or fruit (*see* box right) with plenty of water. Eat little and often to save your digestive system having to work too hard.

Eat when the going gets easy

It is easier to eat and drink when you're riding on the flat and in a straight line; climbing, descending and cornering demand your full concentration. Take advantage of the food served at the rest stops but don't eat anything you haven't previously used in training.

WHAT TO EAT IN THE SADDLE

For rides lasting longer than 90 minutes, you will need food to replenish energy levels. Make sure you also drink plenty of water.

- Energy bars
- Cereal bars, fruit bars and breakfast bars (choose varieties that contain no hydrogenated fat and contain less than 5 g total fat)
- Energy gels
- Bananas and other fruit
- Malt loaf or fruit cake
- Raisins or sultanas
- Fig rolls

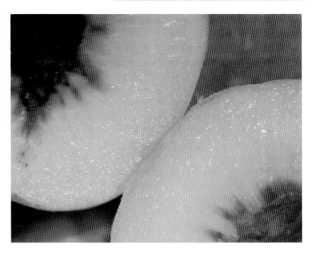

Q&A

Question: *Will flat cola help me keep going longer?*

Answer: Many cyclists swear by drinking flat cola during long rides and races. However, much of the claimed benefits are based on hearsay handed down from one competitor to another. The truth is that cola possesses no special performance-enhancing quality; it is a simply a sugary drink containing around 11 g of sugar per 100 ml – equivalent to two teaspoons of sugar. Cola can give you a quick energy boost but won't hydrate you very fast as it is too concentrated to empty from the stomach quickly. You will get a similar energy boost from an isotonic sports drink, diluted juice, energy gel or solid food taken with a drink of water. Cola also supplies caffeine, but you would need to drink around 1 litre of cola to get an endurance benefit. If you must drink cola, dilute 1 part water with 1–2 parts cola; this will give a better carbohydrate concentration (4–8 per cent) for maximum absorption. Bear in mind that cola is very acidic with the ability to dissolve tooth enamel, so swish water around your mouth afterwards. Better still: opt for plain water during races of less than 60 minutes' duration; for longer races, drink orange juice diluted with equal amounts of water for a 4–8 per cent carbohydrate drink naturally packed with vitamins and minerals.

Question: *How can I avoid the 'bonk'?*

Answer: The 'bonk' is a common problem. It happens when you have used up all the glycogen in your muscles and liver and, therefore, run out of energy. To avoid this, drink sports drinks or eat high-carbohydrate snacks regularly during the ride. Try energy bars, bananas, energy gels and cereal or fruit bars. Aim to consume 30–60 g of carbohydrate per hour – equivalent to:

- one or two bars (depending on the size)
- a couple of gel sachets
- two to four bananas
- 500–1,000 ml of an isotonic sports drink (depending on the strength)
- 1 part fruit juice diluted with 1 part water.

After the race

You will probably feel a great sense of accomplishment when you complete the race and cross the finish line. Before you load up your bike and start back home, however, start rehydrating and refuelling your body. Recovery needs to begin now otherwise you could wake up tomorrow feeling weak and very sore.

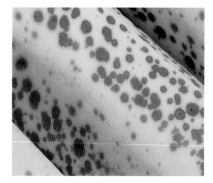

Hit the bottle

Drink plenty of water. As a guide, have a standard (500 ml) water bottle as soon as practical, ideally within the first 30 minutes of finishing the race, then keep drinking small regular amounts until your urine is pale yellow. Again, don't rely on thirst, as this does not tell you whether you are properly rehydrated. If you are dehydrated, a sports drink or diluted juice with a pinch of salt added will deliver fluid faster, and the sodium this contains will help your body retain the fluid better.

Have a bar

Eat a carbohydrate-rich snack within the first 30 minutes of finishing the race; at this time, the blood flow to your muscles is greater and the muscles are more receptive to carbohydrates. This will help re-build glycogen stores. Choose a snack that provides around 1 g of carbohydrate per kilogram of bodyweight. For example, if you weigh 70 kg, you need to eat 70 g of carbohydrate immediately after the race, so try a sports drink or nutrition (sports) bar.

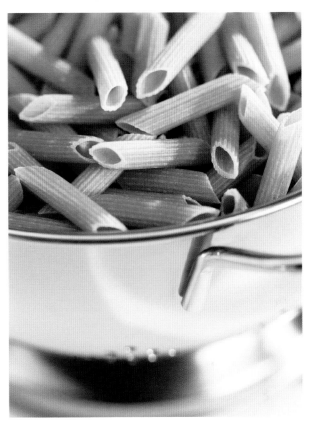

Chow down

Follow your post-race snack with a carbohydrate-rich meal within two hours. Including a small portion of lean protein will help replenish glycogen faster as well as help with muscle repair. Try rice with chicken, pasta with pasta sauce and cheese, a jacket potato with tuna or baked beans on toast.

Pass on the fry-up

It may be tempting to head for the nearest greasy spoon café, burger van or fast food restaurant after a race. But remember: fried, fatty or spicy foods will sit heavily in your stomach, impeding your recovery. Opt for lighter meals and save the greasy stuff for later on if you must!

Swimming galas

The week before the gala

To help you put in your best performance in a swimming gala and recover quicker between heats, ensure that you have normal or 'full' glycogen stores in your muscles. This is especially important if you have several races in one day.

Get out of the pool early

For the last few days before a gala, you should cut back on your swimming training (and other intense activities) then rest completely for the last day or two. This will allow the carbohydrate you eat to be stored as glycogen and not to be burned during a workout.

Stay balanced

Eating a balanced diet is really all you need to do during the week before a gala. Providing you ease back on training, you will allow your muscles to fill out with glycogen. Keep your fat intake low and focus on slow-release (low GI) carbohydrates in your diet. Continue to eat 2–3 portions of protein a day.

Keep drinking

Take care not to become dehydrated during the week before the gala. Check the colour of your urine – it should be pale yellow or almost clear. Aim to drink at least 2 litres of fluids per day, and more in hot weather.

RECOVERY SNACKS

Eat the following with 150–300 ml of water or diluted fruit juice (1 part juice to 1–2 parts water).

- Fruit and yoghurt
- Flapjack
- Cereal bar, sports bar or breakfast bar
- Fruit loaf (*see* recipe on page 192)
- Fruit buns or scones
- Sandwich or bagel with light filling, e.g. turkey, jam, thin cheese slices
- Meal replacement shake
- Milkshake
- Dried fruit and nuts

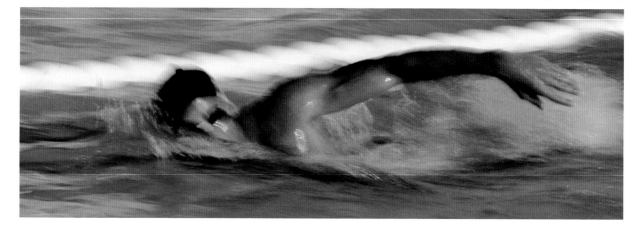

Q&A

Question: *Why do I feel ravenous after swimming?*

Answer: An increased appetite is your body's way of telling you to eat. After a hard workout, you need to replace the fuel you have just used. Your appetite probably seems bigger after swimming than after other activities because you are cooler. Other activities that make you hot for a while after exercise dampen the appetite temporarily.

After swimming, eat a carbohydrate-rich snack (for example, a sandwich, baked potato or fruit and yoghurt) but choose wisely and don't get carried away! There is no evidence that swimmers need to eat any more food after a workout than runners, cyclists or gym-goers. Unfortunately, most of the foods on offer at swimming venues – crisps, chips, chocolate bars, etc. – are not ideal snacks for refuelling. Take your own food to ensure you eat something healthy and nutritious.

Question: *I normally swim first thing in the morning, before breakfast and before work. Am I burning more fat this way or would it be better to eat something before I get to the pool?*

Answer: The answer depends on whether you are swimming primarily to lose weight or to increase fitness. By swimming on an empty stomach you won't necessarily burn more calories but, over time, you could burn more fat. With low insulin levels in your bloodstream, you can theoretically force your body to use more fat for fuel. The downside, though, is that you may run out of energy. If you slow down sooner than you'd like, you could try having a glass of juice, a sports drink, a meal replacement shake or a slice of toast and jam before you start swimming, to boost your intensity and endurance. However, if you have plenty of energy for the early morning swim and you're getting results, stick with what you're doing.

The day before the gala

Keep exercise to a minimum and eat well-balanced meals and snacks. You need to top-up muscle glycogen stores and stay properly hydrated.

Eat little and often

Eat small meals every two to four hours to keep blood sugar levels steady and fuel your muscles in preparation for the event. Avoid big meals or over-eating during the evening, as this will almost certainly make you feel uncomfortable and lethargic the next day.

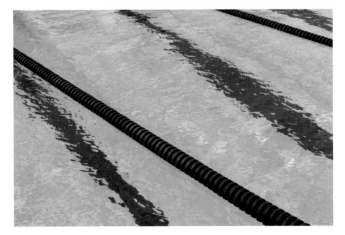

Try liquid meals

If you feel nervous you probably won't have much of an appetite. Try liquid meals such as meal replacement shakes, milkshakes, yoghurt drinks or smoothies. Swimmers sometimes find that semi-liquid or 'slushy' foods are easier to digest when they get pre-race nerves. Try rice pudding, custard, jelly, puréed or tinned fruit, instant porridge (which is smoother than normal porridge oats) or ripe bananas.

Say no to a curry

Avoid eating anything that may cause stomach discomfort. Curries, spicy foods, baked beans and pulses (unless you are used to eating them) can cause gas and bloating. Stick to plain and familiar foods.

Drink water

Keep yourself hydrated by drinking at least 2 litres of water (or equivalent non-caffeinated drinks) throughout the day. Aim to have at least one cup or glass each hour. Your urine should be pale or almost clear.

On the day of the gala

Your aims should be to keep blood sugar levels steady, top-up liver glycogen stores in the morning and stay properly hydrated.

Don't swim on empty

Even if you feel nervous, eat some breakfast. Skipping breakfast can leave you feeling light-headed during your event. As blood sugar levels dip, you'll not only feel weak but fuzzy-headed too, as glucose is your brain's main fuel source. Stick to easily digested foods, for example, cereal with milk, porridge, yoghurt, some fruit or toast with jam. Try a liquid meal if you can't eat solid food. Leave 2–4 hours between eating and swimming.

Check out the fibre

Bran cereals and other fibre-rich foods may cause gas and bowel problems during the event, so it may be better to eat a cereal with a low-fibre content. However, rehearse your pre-swim meal in training so you know exactly what agrees with you.

PRE-EVENT MEALS

- Cereal (low fibre) with fruit and milk
- Porridge with honey
- Meal replacement shake
- Milkshake
- Banana and yoghurt
- Toast with jam or honey
- Smoothie

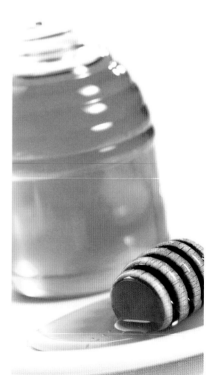

Eat a snack

If you will be racing later in the day, schedule a mini-meal or lunch two to four hours before the start of the race. The meal should be rich in carbohydrate and contain a little protein. Try sandwiches with a lean protein filling, a baked potato with tuna or cheese, a light pasta dish or a meal replacement shake.

Drink two hours before you race

Aim to have 400–600 ml of water, a sports drink or diluted fruit juice during the two hours before the race. This will allow plenty of time for the fluid to be absorbed into the body and for any excess to be excreted. Your urine should be pale yellow in colour by the start of the race.

Nibble between heats

If you will be competing in several heats, you will need to rehydrate and refuel during rest periods. It is best to eat frequent light snacks between heats to keep blood sugar levels constant. Try to eat and drink as soon as possible after your heat, allowing a couple of hours between eating and swimming. Take frequent drinks of water. If you cannot eat solid food, have sports drinks, diluted juice or flavoured milk, to ensure you get the carbohydrate you need.

Pack a lunch box or hamper

If you don't know what food and drink will be available at the venue, take your own. Organise yourself the day before so that you have a supply of suitable foods and drinks for race day. Remember: don't eat anything that you haven't already tried during training.

After the event

Well done for completing the event! Before you begin celebrating, think about rehydrating and refuelling your body – your body will thank you for it the following day!

SNACKS FOR BETWEEN HEATS

- Flavoured milk or milkshake
- Sandwiches, rolls or bagels with low-fat fillings
- Bananas, grapes, apples, oranges
- Dried fruit
- Nuts
- Cereal bars, breakfast bars, fruit bars, sports bars (check they contain no hydrogenated fat)
- Rice cakes
- Mini boxes (variety packs) of cereal

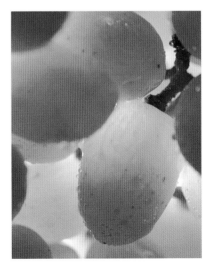

Reach for the bottle

Drink at least 250–500 ml of water as soon as you've got changed, or at least within 30 minutes of finishing your event. If you are dehydrated, with dark coloured and/or a small volume of urine, have a sports drink or diluted juice with a pinch of salt added, to help you rehydrate faster.

Plan a snack

Kick-start your recovery by eating a carbohydrate-rich snack within 30 minutes of completing the event. Glycogen is re-stocked faster than normal for up to two hours after exercise so take advantage of this opportunity to refuel. Aim to consume around 1 g of carbohydrate per kilogram of bodyweight; if you weigh 70 kg, you will need to eat 70 g of carbohydrate. A little protein (1 g of protein for every 3 g of carbohydrate) increases glycogen storage and speeds up the rate of muscle repair. Consume this either in liquid or solid form (*see* box right).

Enjoy a meal

After you have attended to your immediate refuelling needs, you need to plan a balanced meal for about two hours later. It should be high in carbohydrate and contain a little protein and a little (unsaturated) fat. Try pasta with chicken and vegetables, a slice of pizza with salad or a jacket potato with tuna and ratatouille. Avoid the temptation to gorge on fast foods, which could make you feel unwell shortly after an event.

Triathlon events

Much of the advice below is also covered in the sections on running, cycling and swimming.

The week before the event

Your goals are to maximise muscle glycogen stores and keep yourself hydrated.

RECOVERY SNACKS

Eat the following with 150–300 ml of water or diluted fruit juice (1 part juice to 1–2 parts water).

- Cereal bar, sports bar or breakfast bar

- Meal replacement shake and fruit

- Fruit loaf or fruit buns

- Sandwich with lean filing, e.g. chicken, ham, thin cheese slices

- Yoghurt drink

- Smoothie

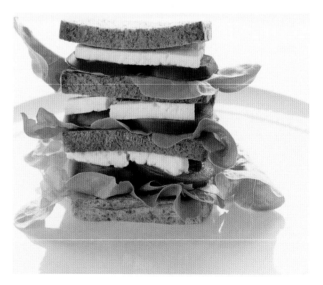

The week before the event

■ *Test in training what you plan to do during the race. Whatever you plan to do during the race, rehearse it in training. Practise drinking from a water bottle on the bike. Or, if you plan to use a camel pack in the event, use it during your training rides. Practise grabbing cups and drinking on the move without spilling or choking. Experiment with different foods – gels, bars, and bananas – to find the types and amounts that suit you best. Research the foods and drinks to be provided at the stations so you can test them out beforehand. Alternatively, take your own supplies.*

■ *Carb up. Tipping the balance a little more in favour of carbohydrates (roughly 60–70 per cent carbohydrate calories) will boost glycogen levels and give you more fuel for the event.*

■ *Taper. Tapering your training along with increasing your carbohydrate intake can increase endurance by as much as 20 per cent.*

■ *Drink enough. Try to drink at least 2 litres of water (or equivalent) each day to ensure you are fully hydrated.*

■ *Eat regular meals and snacks. Dividing your food intake into several medium or small meals and snacks will not only encourage glycogen storage but also avoids stomach discomfort.*

EATING AND DRINKING IN THE SADDLE

■ Many triathletes use specially designed packs containing a plastic bladder (such as a camel pack). This will allow you to carry larger volumes of drink without needing to stop off to refill your bottle.

■ For a cooler drink, add ice cubes to your drink or freeze half the bottle (or camel pack) overnight then top it up before you get on your bike.

■ Carry small snacks in the pockets of your jersey.

■ Wrap dried fruit and biscuits in foil or small re-sealable plastic bags.

■ Soft textured bars may be wrapped around your handlebars for easy access.

■ Practise riding without holding on to the handlebars so that you can balance more easily while you eat and drink.

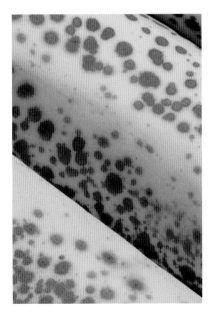

The day before the event

Complete your taper today – perform only very light exercise. Your aim is to top-up muscle glycogen stores and ensure you are properly hydrated.

> **tip** **The day before the event**
>
> - *Little and often. Eat smaller, more frequent meals than usual to maximise glycogen storage.*
> - *Don't try any new foods. Play it safe by sticking to familiar foods. Don't risk an upset stomach – steer away from anything spicy or salty, and avoid meat or fish that may be undercooked.*
> - *Take to the bottle. Keep a water bottle handy so you remember to drink regularly throughout the day. This is especially important if you are travelling to the race venue, as it's easy to forget to drink.*
> - *Beware of the gas. Avoid gas-forming foods (or combinations of food) such as baked beans and other pulses, cruciferous vegetables (broccoli, Brussels sprouts, cauliflower), bran cereals and spicy foods the night before the race. These can make you feel uncomfortable.*
> - *Don't over-indulge. Keep your supper light otherwise you risk feeling heavy and sluggish the next day. If you must drink alcohol, limit yourself to one or two units (one pint of ordinary strength lager), otherwise you risk dehydration.*

The day of the event

All that remains to be done before the race is to top–up liver glycogen stores at breakfast time (liver glycogen is normally depleted during the overnight fast), replace any fluids lost overnight and keep blood sugar levels steady.

> **tip** **The day of the event**
>
> - *Get organised. Don't rely on finding nutritious foods at outlets en route or at the venue – healthy choices are often limited at these places. It is always best to take your own food supplies for the journey as well as for race day. Take extra water in case of delays.*
> - *Eat breakfast. Eat a moderate-sized carbohydrate-based pre-event meal about 2–3 hours before competing. It should also be low in fat and contain a little protein. Try porridge, toast, cereal, fruit or yoghurt.*
> - *Drink. Aim to drink 400–600 ml of water, a sports drink or diluted fruit juice (1 part juice to 1–2 parts water) during the two-hour period before the race. Your urine should be a very pale yellow.*

PRE-RACE MEALS

- Porridge with fruit and honey
- Cereal with milk and yoghurt
- Scrambled egg on toast
- Toast with honey plus yoghurt or a milky drink
- Smoothie made with fruit and yoghurt

During the race

Drink regularly

You will not be able to drink during the swim but start drinking as soon as you get on the bike. Your goal is then to continue drinking little and often, aiming for 150–350 ml every 15 to 20 minutes. Two or three gulps at a time suits many triathletes. Stick to whatever fluids you drank during your training. Remember that wind-chill and rapid evaporation of sweat can mask feelings of dehydration.

Fuel in the saddle

For events longer than 90 minutes, you will need to consume extra carbohydrates in the form of sports drinks, energy gels, bars or fruit; these should be taken with plenty of water to maintain blood sugar levels. Take advantage of the food served at the rest stops but don't eat anything you haven't previously eaten in training.

Eat on the flat

It is easier to eat and drink when you're riding on the flat and in a straight line; climbing, descending and cornering demand your full concentration.

Q&A

Question: *Ironmen can spend hours in the saddle and often complain of becoming sick of sweet foods. Are there any savoury foods that would be a suitable replacement?*

Answer: If you prefer savoury foods, try rolls, bagels, sandwiches, rice cakes and crackers. Soup is also a good choice because it provides vital fluid, but try to have homemade instead of ready-bought varieties, which can be very high in salt.

After the race

The key to fast recovery is food and drink, so the sooner you eat and drink the better.

WHAT TO EAT IN THE SADDLE

- Energy bars, cereal bars, fruit bars and breakfast bars
- Energy gels
- Bananas and other fruit
- Malt loaf or fruit cake
- Raisins or sultanas
- Fig rolls

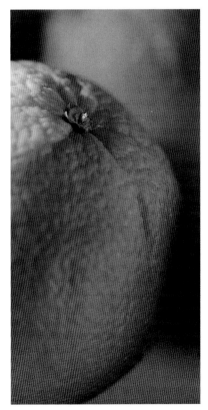

Mine's a pint

Make sure you are rehydrated before embarking on a celebratory drink. When drinking alcohol, the best choices are lager, beer and shandy (the extra fluid will reduce further dehydration) – or alternate water with an alcoholic drink.

Drink, drink, drink

You should drink 500 ml of water within the first 30 minutes of completing the event then keep drinking small regular amounts until your urine is pale in colour. If you are dehydrated, a sports drink or diluted juice with a pinch of salt added will deliver fluid faster, and the sodium they contain will help your body retain the fluid better.

Grab a snack

Eat a carbohydrate-rich snack within the first 30 minutes of completing the event, when blood flow to the muscles is greater and glycogen storage is one and a half times faster than normal.

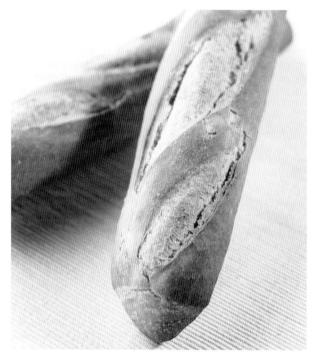

Eat wisely

Eat a carbohydrate-rich meal within two hours of finishing the race. This should also include a portion of lean protein, to help replenish glycogen faster and aid muscle repair. Opt for light meals such as:

- pasta with tomato sauce
- a jacket potato with tuna or cottage cheese
- chicken sandwiches
- a bagel with a little cheese
- a vegetable and tofu stir-fry
- noodles with prawns.

Avoid fast food

Resist the temptation to eat fast or junk food after a race. Just because the race is over, doesn't mean that you should load your system with fat, sugar and salt. Burgers, chips, kebabs and curries will sit heavily in your stomach at this time, impeding your recovery.

Football and rugby matches

The week before the match

A football or rugby game heavily taxes your muscle glycogen levels so you need to make sure you have plenty in reserve. Build them up the week before the match by eating extra carbohydrate and tapering your training. A good nutritional strategy will ensure you are match fit on the day.

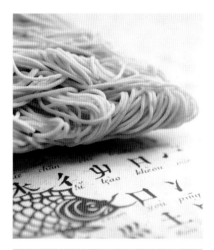

Taper and carb up

Reduce the amount and intensity of training a few days before your match. During this time you should also boost your carbohydrate intake (aim for 7–10 g of carbohydrates per 1 kg of body weight); to keep calorie input constant, reduce the amount of saturated fat you consume. This will ensure that your muscles are fully stocked with glycogen and your body stays lean.

Graze

Eat two or three high-carbohydrate snacks in addition to three regular meals to help you carry out your carbohydrate-loading plan. This will also be easier on the digestive system and stop you feeling bloated.

Drink more water

It is important to drink plenty of fluids in the pre-match week – dehydration is cumulative and can hinder your performance. Aim for 2 litres of water (or equivalent) each day.

The day before the match

Plan to rest today so that you do not deplete glycogen stores. You should also aim to top-up glycogen stores and stay well-hydrated.

POST-RACE RECOVERY SNACKS

- Yoghurt drink
- Dried fruit and nuts
- Chocolate-coated raisins and nuts
- Fresh fruit and yoghurt
- Flapjack
- Cereal bar, sports bar or breakfast bar
- Fruit cake or malt loaf
- Sandwich with peanut butter or cheese
- Meal replacement (carbohydrate and protein) shake
- Flavoured milk or milkshake

The day before the match

- *Eat little and often throughout the day. Divide your food intake into several small meals and snacks and avoid eating big meals. This will encourage your muscles to turn all the carbohydrates you eat into glycogen.*
- *Don't pig out. Big meals the night before will sit heavily in your stomach and probably keep you awake at night. You may also feel sluggish the next day.*
- *Stick with familiar foods. Opt for plain and simple foods otherwise you risk an upset stomach on match day. If travelling to a match, find out what food will be provided in advance and be prepared to take your own supplies.*
- *Keep a water bottle handy. Remember to drink regularly throughout the day, especially if you are travelling.*

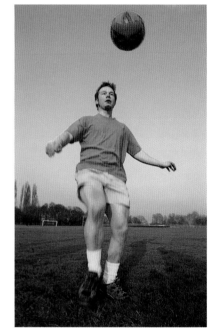

On match day

By now, your muscle glycogen stores should be fully stocked. All that remains to be done before the race is to replenish liver glycogen stores following the overnight fast and keep blood sugar levels up.

Plan your pre-match meal

Aim to eat between two and four hours before kick-off. Your pre-match meal should be high in carbohydrate with a small amount of protein and healthy fat to provide sustained energy; aim for approximately 500–600 calories. Try porridge, pancakes, cereal or toast with yoghurt and fruit before a morning match. Pasta with chicken or rice with beans or fish would be a good choice before an afternoon match.

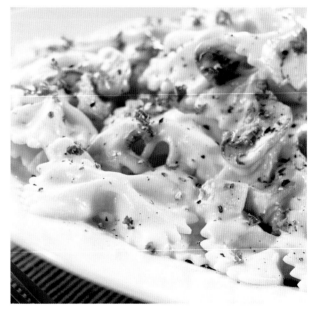

Drink right

During the two hours before the match, drink at least 500 ml of water or, ideally, a sports drink containing 6 g of carbohydrate per 100 ml or diluted fruit juice (equal parts juice and water). Then drink another 125–250 ml just before kick-off.

During the match

Drink at every opportunity

Swig a sports drink (6 g of carbohydrate per 100 ml) or diluted juice (equal parts juice and water) at half-time and during injury time-outs. This will help avoid dehydration – you can lose 2 litres of fluid (or more) through sweating during a match, according to various studies. Such losses can reduce running performance and increase fatigue.

Choose the right drink

Stick with whichever drink you have used in training and don't try anything new. UK researchers found that players swigging a sports drink during a game allowed fewer goals and scored significantly more times, especially during the second half, than those who drank flavoured water (placebo).

After the match

The game may be over but your recovery strategy starts now. This is important if you want to train or have enough energy to move about in the next few days.

Replace fluid

Start drinking as soon as possible after the match, i.e. before you shower. It is vital that you begin to replace the fluid you've lost. Try to drink around 500 ml of a sports drink or diluted juice in the first 30 minutes after the match, little and often, then keep gulping every 5 or 10 minutes until you are passing clear urine.

Hold the beer

Make sure you are rehydrated before embarking on a celebratory drink. The best alcoholic drinks are lager, beer and shandy (the extra fluid will reduce further dehydration) – or alternate water with an alcoholic drink.

PRE-MATCH MEALS

Eat the following with 150–300 ml of water or diluted fruit juice (1 part juice to 1–2 parts water).

- Porridge with raisins and honey
- Cereal with milk and bananas
- Toast with jam and a milky drink
- Pancakes or waffles with honey
- Pasta with chicken and salad
- Rice with beans or grilled fish and vegetables
- Spaghetti Bolognese with vegetables

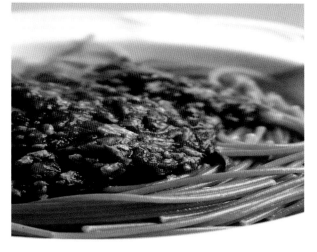

Grab a snack

The match will have depleted glycogen stores in your leg muscles, so your mission is to restock those stores immediately. Eat a high-carbohydrate snack (1 g of carbohydrate per 1 kg of bodyweight) within the first 30–60 minutes of the match ending. This can be solid food or a drink – whatever feels right. Including a little protein with the carbohydrate (approx 1 part protein to 3 parts carbohydrate) will speed glycogen recovery.

Don't pig out!

Resist the temptation to celebrate your match result with fatty foods and alcohol. Burgers, chips, kebabs and curries will sit heavily on the stomach, slow your recovery and leave you feeling bloated and sluggish. Choose plainer options, for example, noodles, rice dishes or cheese and tomato pizza, or smaller portions with extra vegetables.

POST-MATCH MEALS

- Pasta with tomato pasta sauce, cheese and vegetables
- Jacket potato with tuna, sweetcorn and salad
- Chicken with roast vegetables and rice
- Turkey and vegetable kebabs with pitta bread
- Baked or grilled salmon, rice and salad

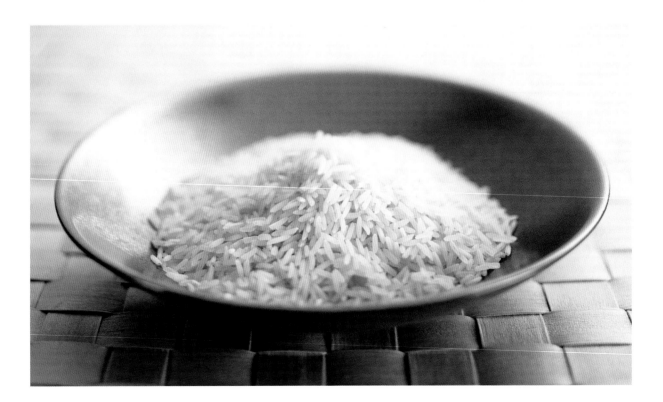

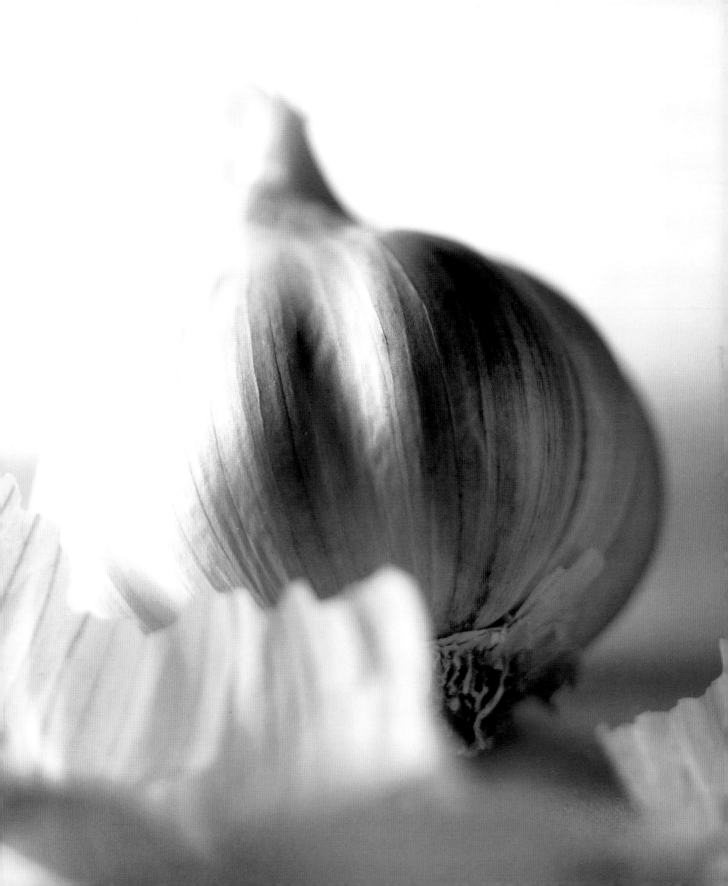

10

recipe file

Power porridge

Starting the day with a bowl of porridge gives you a fantastic energy boost. Add chopped fresh fruit, such as sliced banana, blueberries or strawberries or dried fruit to boost the fibre and vitamin content.

MAKES 1 LARGE SERVING

- 60 g (2 oz.) porridge oats
- 350 ml (12 fl oz.) skimmed milk
- 25 g (1 oz.) raisins, dates or figs
- 1 banana, sliced
- 2 tsp honey or maple syrup

1 *Mix the oats and milk.*
2 *Cook in a microwave for approximately 4 minutes, stirring halfway through, or in a saucepan for approximately 5 minutes, stirring continuously.*
3 *Add the raisins and banana and extra milk if desired.*
4 *Spoon on the honey or maple syrup.*

Muesli with fruit and nuts

This muesli is very easy to make. I like to soak the oats overnight – they're nicer when they're soft and have absorbed the flavours of the dried fruit. Oats are rich in soluble fibre, which helps regulate blood sugar and insulin levels as well as reduce cholesterol levels. They also supply B vitamins, iron, magnesium and zinc. Nuts are rich in vitamin E, essential fatty acids and protein.

MAKES 2 SERVINGS

- 85 g (3 oz.) porridge oats
- 150 ml (¼ pt.) skimmed, soya, rice, almond or oat 'milk'
- 2 tbsp raisins (or other dried fruit such as figs)
- 2 tbsp chopped brazils or walnuts
- 1 tbsp ground linseeds (optional)
- 125 g (4 oz.) blueberries, raspberries or strawberries

1 *In a large bowl, mix together the oats (or other flakes), milk, dried fruit, nuts and ground linseeds. Cover and leave overnight in the fridge.*
2 *Serve in individual bowls, topped with the fresh berries.*

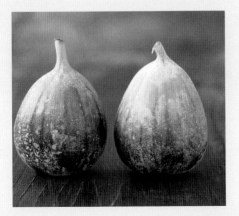

Granola

Oats are rich in soluble fibre and provide slow-release energy as well as plenty of B vitamins and iron. Almonds and hazelnuts supply protein, calcium, zinc and healthy monounsaturated oils.

MAKES 4 SERVINGS

- 225 g (8 oz.) oats
- 60 g (2 oz.) sunflower seeds
- 60 g (2 oz.) flaked almonds
- 60 g (2 oz.) hazelnuts, crushed
- 2 tbsp clear honey
- 2 tbsp rapeseed oil
- 85 ml (3 fl oz.) water
- 1 tsp vanilla extract
- 1 tsp ground cinnamon
- 1 tsp ground ginger
- a pinch of ground allspice (optional)
- 85 g (3 oz.) chopped dates, raisins or apricots (or a mixture)

1 *Heat the oven to 190°C/375°F/Gas mark 5.*
2 *Mix the oats, sunflower seeds, almonds and hazelnuts together in a bowl.*
3 *In a separate bowl, combine the honey, oil, water, vanilla and spices. Add to the oat mixture and mix well.*
4 *Spread out on a nonstick baking tray and bake in the oven for 30–40 minutes, stirring occasionally until evenly browned.*
5 *Cool and then mix in the dried fruit. Store in an airtight container.*
6 *Serve with skimmed, soya, rice or oat milk, natural yoghurt and/or fresh fruit.*

Breakfast bars

For a fibre boost, try these simple bars. They are low in fat and packed with B vitamins and beta-carotene.

MAKES 12 BARS

- 125 g (4 oz.) ready-to-eat apricots, chopped
- 125 g (4 oz.) dates, chopped
- 1 egg
- 1 tbsp oil
- 125 ml (4 fl oz.) plain yogurt
- 60 g (2 oz.) sugar
- 60 g (2 oz.) self-raising wholemeal flour
- 4 Weetabix, crumbled

1 *Combine the apricots, dates, egg, oil and yogurt in a bowl. Mix well. Stir in the sugar, flour and Weetabix. Add a little milk if the mixture is too stiff.*
2 *Spoon into a lightly oiled nonstick 20 cm (8 in.) square baking dish.*
3 *Bake at 180 °C/375 °F/Gas mark 5 for 20–25 minutes.*
4 *Cool and cut into bars.*

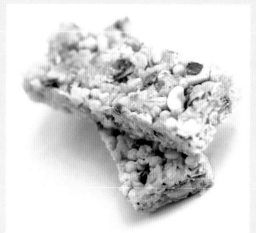

Breakfast muffins

These tasty low-fat muffins are ideal for eating on the move.

MAKES 12 MUFFINS

- 125 g (4 oz.) white self-raising flour
- 125 g (4 oz.) wholemeal self-raising flour
- 1 tbsp oil
- 40 g (1.5 oz.) soft brown sugar
- 1 egg
- 150 ml (5 fl oz.) skimmed milk
- 60 g (2 oz.) dried fruit

1 *Preheat the oven to 220 °C/425 °F/Gas mark 7.*
2 *Mix the flours together in a bowl. Add the oil, sugar, egg and milk. Mix well. Stir in the dried fruit.*
3 *Spoon into a nonstick muffin tray and bake for approximately 15 minutes until golden brown.*

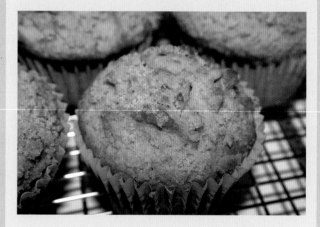

Breakfast pancakes with fruit

The eggs and milk in pancakes are good sources of protein. Milk is also rich in calcium, while the fruit fillings provide vitamin C, beta-carotene and fibre.

MAKES 6

- 70 g (2.5 oz.) plain white flour
- 70 g (2.5 oz.) plain wholemeal flour
- 1 egg
- 300 ml (½ pt.) skimmed milk
- A little vegetable oil or oil spray for frying

Filling:
- Sliced bananas, sliced strawberries, apple puree with raisins, lightly crushed raspberries, frozen berry mixture (thawed), chopped mango, or sliced nectarines or peaches
- Natural bio-yoghurt, to serve

1 *Place all of the pancake ingredients in a liquidiser and blend until smooth.*
   Alternatively mix the flours in a bowl. Make a well in the centre. Beat the egg and milk and gradually add to the flour, beating to make a smooth batter.
2 *Place a nonstick frying pan over a high heat. Spray with oil spray or add a few drops of oil.*
3 *Pour in enough batter to coat the pan thinly and cook for 1–2 minutes until golden brown on the underside.*
4 *Turn the pancake and cook the other side for 30–60 seconds.*
5 *Turn out on to a plate, cover and keep warm while you make the other pancakes.*
6 *Serve with any of the suggested fresh fruit fillings and bio-yoghurt.*

Oatmeal and raisin scotch pancakes

A fantastic way to start the day, these pancakes give you slow release complex carbs, protein and soluble fibre. Alternatively, they make nutritious snacks that you can wrap and pop in your kit bag.

MAKES 8 PANCAKES

- 2 large eggs
- 225 g (8 oz.) cottage cheese
- 1 tbsp margarine or low-fat spread
- 125 g (4 oz.) oatmeal or porridge oats
- 85 g (3 oz.) raisins or currants

1 *Place the eggs, cottage cheese, margarine and oatmeal in a liquidiser and blend until smooth. Alternatively, beat together in a bowl.*
2 *Carefully stir in the raisins or currants.*
3 *Lightly brush a nonstick frying pan with oil. Drop tablespoons of the batter onto the hot pan. When bubbles appear on the surface, flip over and cook one minute more.*
4 *Serve with fresh fruit, pureed fruit or honey.*

SOUP

Vegetable stock

Use this stock for making soups, stews and casseroles in any recipes that call for stock. Alternatively, use 4 tsp low-sodium vegetable bouillon powder dissolved in 1 l (2 pt.) of hot water.

MAKES 600 ML (1 PT.)

- 900 ml (1.5 pt.) water
- 2 onions, sliced
- 2 carrots, roughly sliced
- 2 celery sticks, halved
- 1 leek, halved
- 2 bay leaves
- 2 sprigs of thyme
- 2 sprigs of parsley
- 8 black peppercorns
- Pinch of sea salt to season

1 Put the water, vegetables, herbs and seasonings in a large saucepan.
2 Bring to the boil and simmer gently for at least 1 hour. Leave to cool and then strain.

A–Z vegetable soup

MAKES 4 SERVINGS

Possibly the easiest soup ever, you can vary this soup endlessly according to which seasonal vegetables you have to hand. In any case, you're guaranteed a tasty and speedy vitamin feast.

MAKES

- 1 onion, chopped
- 1 garlic clove, crushed
- 1 l (1¾ pt) vegetable stock (home-made or vegetable bouillon powder dissolved in boiling water)
- 750 g (1.5 lb.) vegetables of your choice (see below)
- 1 tbsp olive oil
- Season with salt and freshly ground black pepper
- 1 tbsp fresh mixed herbs, e.g. chives, parsely, marjorum (or 1 tsp (dried herbs)

Vegetables:
- Chopped potato, sliced courgettes, sliced carrots, diced pumpkin, chopped green beans, frozen peas, broccoli florets, cauliflower florets

1 *Place the onion, garlic, olive oil, vegetable stock and vegetables in a large saucepan. Bring to the boil and simmer for approximately 20 minutes or until the vegetables are soft.*
2 *Turn off the heat. Add the olive oil, seasoning, and herbs.*
3 *For a smooth soup, liquidise in a blender or food processor or hand blender. For a chunky thick soup, liquidise half the soup and return to the pan.*

Minestrone soup

Packed with fibre, potassium, vitamin C (from the tinned tomatoes, leeks and courgettes) and beta-carotene (from the carrots), this soup is almost a complete meal. The haricot beans are good sources of protein, complex carbohydrate and soluble fibre, while the pasta provides extra carbs.

MAKES 4 SERVINGS

- 1 litre (1¾ pints) vegetable stock
- 1 onion, chopped
- 2 garlic cloves, crushed
- 2 carrots, chopped
- 1 medium potato, peeled and diced
- 1 leeks, trimmed and thinly sliced
- 2 tsp dried basil
- 420 g (14 oz.) tinned haricot, cannelini or flageolet beans
- 2 small courgettes, trimmed and sliced
- 125 g (4 oz.) fine green beans
- 125 g (4 oz.) small wheat-free pasta shapes
- 400 g (14 oz.) tinned chopped tomatoes

1 *Pour the vegetable stock into a large saucepan. Bring to the boil and add the onion, garlic, carrots, potatoes, leeks, basil and haricot beans. Lower the heat, cover and simmer for 15 minutes until the vegetables are tender.*
2 *Add the courgettes, green beans, tomatoes and pasta and continue cooking for a further 5 minutes or until the pasta is just cooked (check the cooking instructions on the packet).*
3 *Serve the soup hot in individual bowls with lots of freshly grated Parmesan cheese.*

Thai chicken and coconut

Chicken is rich in protein and B vitamins. The ginger and chillies stimulate the immune system.

MAKES 4 SERVINGS

- 2 chicken breasts cut into strips
- Zest and juice of 1 lime
- 400 ml (14 fl oz.) coconut milk
- 400 ml (14 fl oz.) hot chicken or vegetable stock
- 1 stem lemon grass, cut into strips
- 2.5 cm (1 in.) fresh ginger, peeled and grated
- 1 red chilli, finely chopped (optional)
- 2 tbsp chopped fresh coriander leaves

1 *In a shallow dish, sprinkle the lime juice over the chicken pieces, cover and leave to marinate in the fridge for at least 30 minutes.*

2 *Place the remaining ingredients in a large saucepan and heat until boiling.*

3 *Add the chicken pieces and lime juice. Reduce the heat and simmer for 15 minutes.*

4 *Ladle into four bowls and sprinkle over the coriander leaves.*

Leek and potato soup

Perfect winter fodder, this soup makes use of seasonal vegetables. Leeks are rich in fibre and the green part in particular provides folate, vitamin E, iron, beta-carotene and vitamin C.

MAKES 4 SERVINGS

- 1 l (1¾ pt.) vegetable stock
- 3 medium potatoes, scrubbed and roughly chopped
- 3 large leeks, sliced
- 1 large carrot, sliced
- a little low-sodium salt and freshly ground black pepper
- a small handful of chopped fresh parsley

1 *Place the vegetable stock, potatoes, leeks and carrots in a large saucepan.*

2 *Bring to the boil, lower the heat, cover and simmer for approximately 20 minutes until the vegetables are tender.*

3 *Remove from the heat and liquidise until smooth using a blender, food processor or a hand blender.*

4 *Return to the saucepan to heat through. Season the soup with the low-sodium salt and freshly ground black pepper. Stir in the fresh parsley.*

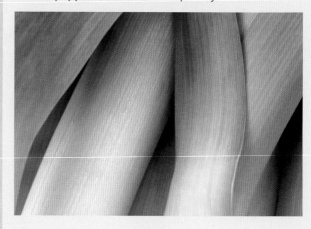

Broccoli and bean soup

This sounds like an unusual combination but it works really well. The mild- flavoured flageolet beans and potato give the soup a creamy texture. Broccoli is one of the most nutritious vegetables, full of vitamin C, iron, folic acid and cancer-fighting phytochemicals.

MAKES 4 SERVINGS

- 4 spring onions, sliced
- 1 garlic clove, crushed
- 2 tsp mild curry powder
- 1.5 l (3 pt.) vegetable stock (or water plus 2 stock cubes)
- 1 medium potato, chopped
- 450 g (1 lb.) broccoli florets
- 1 420 g tin (15 oz.) flageolet beans, drained

1 *Place the onions, garlic and curry powder in a saucepan with about 150 ml ($^1/_4$ pt.) of the stock. Bring to the boil and simmer for approximately 5 minutes.*
2 *Add the remaining stock, the potato and broccoli and simmer for 15–20 minutes.*
3 *Add the beans then purée the soup in a blender or food processor (in small batches if necessary).*

Carrot soup with fresh coriander

This is one of the easiest vegetable soups to make and packed with vital beta-carotene, a powerful antioxidant that helps combat free radicals that cause cancer. It's a firm winter favourite with my family.

MAKES 2 SERVINGS

- 1 tbsp extra virgin olive oil
- 1 small onion, finely sliced
- 1 garlic clove, crushed
- 4 large carrots, sliced
- 500 ml (16 fl oz.) vegetable stock
- 1 bay leaf
- a little low-sodium salt and freshly ground black pepper
- a handful of fresh coriander, roughly chopped

1 *Heat the olive oil in a heavy-based saucepan over a moderate heat. Add the onion and sauté gently for approximately 5 minutes until it is translucent.*
2 *Add the garlic and cook for a further 1–2 minutes. Add the carrots, stock and bay leaf to the pan, stir, and then bring to the boil. Simmer for 15 minutes or until the vegetables are tender.*
3 *Allow the soup to cool slightly for a couple of minutes. Remove and discard the bay leaf.*
4 *Liquidise the soup using a hand or conventional blender. Season to taste with low-sodium salt and pepper, then stir in the fresh coriander.*

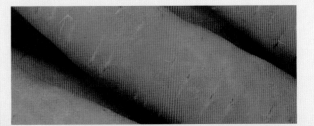

Spicy lentil soup

This soup provides a powerhouse of nutrients. Lentils provide lots of protein as well as complex carbohydrates, fibre, iron, B vitamins, zinc, and selenium. You can add extra vegetables, such as carrots and mushrooms, to boost the nutritional and fibre value.

MAKES 2 SERVINGS

- 1–2 tsp curry paste
- 1 onion, chopped
- 1 garlic clove, crushed
- 2 cm (1 in.) piece root ginger, peeled and finely chopped
- 125 g (4 oz.) red lentils
- 500 ml (16 fl oz.) vegetable stock
- Grated zest and juice of 1 lime
- A little low-sodium salt and freshly ground black pepper
- Chopped fresh mint to garnish

1 *Place the curry paste, onion, garlic and ginger in a large pan and cook gently for 3 minutes.*
2 *Add the lentils and vegetable stock and bring to the boil. Reduce the heat and simmer for 20 minutes.*
3 *Add the lime zest and juice, bring back to the boil and simmer for a further 10 minutes until the lentils are soft. Season to taste with low-sodium salt and pepper.*
4 *Ladle into bowls and garnish with the mint leaves.*

Butternut squash and carrot soup

This soup is really warming and tasty, perfect served with a slice of crusty wholewheat or rye bread. Butternut squash and carrots are rich in beta-carotene, which can help combat premature ageing, heart disease and cancer. Butternut squash is also a useful source of the antioxidant vitamin C, which is needed for immunity and speedy recovery after exercise.

MAKES 2 SERVINGS

- 1 small onion
- ½ medium butternut squash
- 2 carrots, sliced
- 1 garlic clove, crushed
- 1 tsp grated fresh ginger
- Pinch of freshly grated nutmeg (optional)
- 500 ml (16 fl oz.) vegetable stock
- 1 tbsp omega 3-rich oil or extra virgin olive oil
- A little low-sodium salt and freshly ground black pepper

1 *Peel and chop the onion. Peel the butternut squash and cut the flesh into chunks.*
2 *Place the vegetables, garlic, and grated ginger, optional nutmeg and vegetable stock in a large saucepan. Bring to the boil, lower the heat, cover and simmer for approximately 20 minutes until the vegetables are tender.*
3 *Remove from the heat and liquidise with the oil until smooth using a blender, food processor or a hand blender.*
4 *Return to the saucepan to heat through. Season the soup with the low-sodium salt and freshly ground black pepper.*

Turkey and vegetable soup with split peas and barley

This nutritious soup is perfect for fuelling your muscles before a hard workout. Eat 3–4 hours before exercise for a steady blood sugar rise, rather than a rapid surge, minimising the risk of hypoglycaemia (low blood sugar levels) during your workout.

MAKES 4 SERVINGS

- 85 g (3 oz.) green or yellow split peas, soaked overnight in double their volume of water
- 1 l (1¾ pt.) vegetable stock
- 1 onion, chopped
- 2 garlic cloves, crushed
- 2 carrots, chopped
- 1 medium potato, peeled and diced
- 1 leek, trimmed and thinly sliced
- 1 tsp dried thyme
- 40 g (1 ½ oz.) pearl barley
- 2 small courgettes, trimmed and sliced
- 125 g (4 oz.) fine green beans
- 125 g (4 oz.) cooked turkey, cut into chunks
- Freshly ground black pepper
- *To serve:* Grated Parmesan cheese

1 Drain the split peas and place in a saucepan with cold water to cover. Bring to the boil and simmer for 10 minutes. Drain then discard the liquid.
2 Pour the vegetable stock into a large saucepan. Bring to the boil and add the split peas, onion, garlic, carrots, potatoes, leeks, thyme and pearl barley. Lower the heat, cover and simmer for 15 minutes until the vegetables are tender.
3 Add the courgettes, green beans and turkey and continue cooking for a further 5 minutes.
4 Season with the black pepper and serve the soup hot in individual bowls with grated Parmesan cheese.

Baked bean and vegetable soup

This tasty low GI soup is rich in fibre, potassium, vitamin A and fibre. The beans also supply protein, B vitamins and complex carbohydrate. You can substitute other varieties of tinned beans, such as cannelloni or borlotti beans, if you wish.

SERVES 4

- 1 tbsp oil
- 1 onion, chopped
- 1 celery stick, chopped
- 2 carrots, sliced
- 1 clove garlic, crushed
- 1 turnip, chopped
- 1 420 g (15 oz.) tin baked beans
- 75 g (3 oz.) frozen green beans or peas
- 0.5 l (1 ¼ pt.) vegetable stock
- 2 tbsp parsley, chopped

1 Heat the oil in a large saucepan, add the onion and fry until softened.
2 Add the celery, carrots, garlic and turnip. Cover and cook for 5 minutes.
3 Add the baked beans, green beans, and stock . Cover and simmer for 10 minutes until the vegetables are tender.
4 Stir in the parsley. Serve with crusty white bread, French bread or ciabatta bread.

Chicken and mushroom soup

This soup is perfect for using up leftover cooked chicken. It is packed with protein, B vitamins and complex carbs – a great refuelling meal after a tough workout.

MAKES 4 SERVINGS

- 1 l (2 pt.) chicken stock
- 125 g (4 oz.) mushrooms, sliced
- 175 g (6 oz.) lean cooked chicken, skinned and chopped
- 125 g (4 oz.) small pasta shapes
- ½ tsp dried mixed herbs
- Freshly ground black pepper

1 *Put the stock in a large saucepan. Bring to the boil.*
2 *Add the mushrooms, chicken and pasta. Stir well and add the herbs. Cover the pan and simmer for approximately 5 minutes.*
3 *Season with the black pepper and serve with a warm wholemeal roll.*

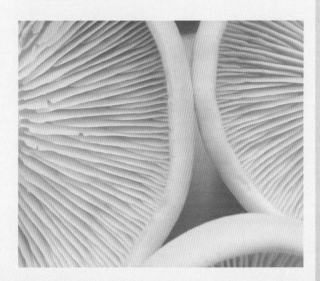

Root vegetable soup

Carrots are super-rich in beta-carotene, a powerful antioxidant that helps prevent cancer, beat premature ageing and promote healthy skin. Parsnips provide good amounts of vitamin E and swede is a good source of vitamin C.

MAKES 4 SERVINGS

- 1 tbsp extra virgin olive oil
- 1 onion, finely sliced
- 450 g (1 lb.) (approximately 6) carrots, sliced
- 225 g (8 oz.) (approximately 2) parsnips, diced
- 225 g (8 oz.) swede, diced
- 1 l (1¾ pt.) vegetable stock
- 1 bay leaf
- A little salt and freshly ground black pepper

1 *Heat the olive oil in a heavy-based saucepan over a moderate heat. Add the onion and sauté gently for approximately 5 minutes until it is translucent.*
2 *Add the carrots, parsnips and swede to the pan and mix well. Cook gently over a moderately low heat for 5 minutes, stirring occasionally, until the vegetables soften a little.*
3 *Add the stock and bay leaf and bring to the boil. Simmer for 15 minutes or until the vegetables are tender.*
4 *Allow the soup to cool slightly for several minutes. Remove and discard the bay leaf. Liquidise the soup using a hand or conventional blender.*

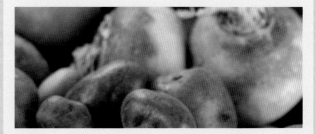

SALADS

SALAD DRESSINGS

Pasta salad

This basic recipe can be infinitely varied according to what vegetables you have at hand. Cold left over cooked vegetables (e.g. carrots, broccoli peas) are also suitable.

MAKES 4 SERVINGS

- 125 g (4 oz.) (1¼ mugs) pasta shells
- ½ red pepper
- ½ yellow pepper
- 60 g (2 oz.) raisins
- 200 g (7 oz.) (approx ½ tin) canned red kidney beans (drained) OR chopped cold chicken OR turkey OR canned tuna
- 2 tomatoes, sliced
- 1 apple, sliced
- 3 tbsp low-fat mayonnaise

1 *Cook the pasta shells according to directions on the packet. Drain and allow to cool.*
2 *Mix the pasta with the peppers, raisins, beans/ chicken/ tuna, tomatoes and apple slices. Combine with the low-fat mayonnaise.*

Coleslaw with almonds

Cabbage is rich in fibre, vitamin C and cancer-protective nutrients called glucosinolates. Carrots are super-rich in beta-carotene, a powerful antioxidant that helps fight cancer.

MAKES 4 SERVINGS

- 4 tbsp natural bio-yoghurt
- 2 tsp Dijon mustard
- 2 tsp low-fat mayonnaise
- 2 tsp lemon juice
- 1 small white cabbage, shredded
- 4 medium carrots, grated
- 1 red onion, thinly sliced
- 30 g (1 oz.) flaked toasted almonds

1 *In a large bowl whisk together the yoghurt, mustard, mayonnaise and lemon juice.*
2 *Add the cabbage, carrots, red onion and almonds, tossing to combine well.*

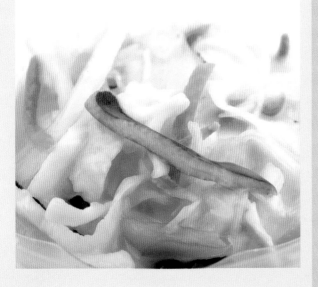

Mixed bean salad

This salad is a great way of boosting your protein intake. Beans also provide soluble fibre, which is great for cleansing the digestive system, as well as B vitamins, iron and zinc.

MAKES 4 SERVINGS

- 85 g (3 oz.) green beans, trimmed and halved
- 225 g (8 oz.) can red kidney beans, drained
- 225 g (8 oz.) can butter beans, drained
- 225 g (8 oz.) can flageolet beans, drained
- 60 g (2 oz.) button mushrooms, sliced
- 2 tbsp extra virgin olive oil
- 1 tsp wholegrain mustard
- 1 tsp clear honey
- 2 tsp cider vinegar
- 1 tbsp fresh parsley, chopped

1 *Steam the green beans for 4–5 minutes. Drain and refresh under cold running water.*
2 *Place the canned beans, green beans and mushrooms in a large bowl and mix together.*
3 *Put the olive oil, mustard, honey, vinegar and parsley in a screw top glass jar, shake well and pour the dressing over the salad.*
4 *Toss lightly and serve. This salad can be kept in the fridge for up to 2 days.*

Potato salad with spinach

New potatoes contain one and a half times more vitamin C than old potatoes. Cook them in a steamer or plunge into fast-boiling water to minimise vitamin losses. Spinach leaves add extra iron and folic acid, as well as delicious flavour.

MAKES 4 SERVINGS

- 900 g (2 lb.) new potatoes, washed
- 4 spring onions, chopped
- Handful of fresh herbs: mint; dill; parsley
- 2 tbsp yogurt
- 2 tbsp salad cream or reduced fat mayonnaise
- 125 g (4 oz.) baby spinach leaves

1 *Cook the potatoes in boiling water until tender. Drain. Halve any large ones.*
2 *Combine the onions, herbs, yogurt and salad cream or mayonnaise in a large bowl.*
3 *Mix with the potatoes and spinach leaves.*

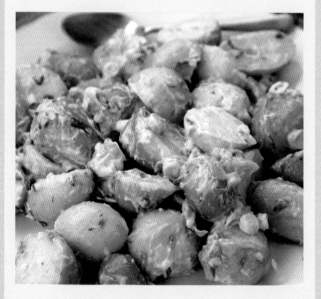

Bean and tuna salad

This protein-packed salad is perfect for refuelling after an intense workout. Beans are rich sources of iron and zinc, as well as fibre for keeping your digestive system healthy.

MAKES 4 SERVINGS

- 2 tins (2 × 420 g/15 oz.) cannelini or red kidney beans, drained
- 2 celery sticks, chopped
- 200 g (7 oz.) tinned tuna
- 125 g (4 oz.) green beans, cooked
- 2 tbsp red wine vinegar
- 1 tsp olive oil
- Handful of fresh herbs: chives; parsley

1 *Combine the beans, celery, tuna and green beans in a bowl.*
2 *Mix together the vinegar, oil and herbs and combine with the salad.*

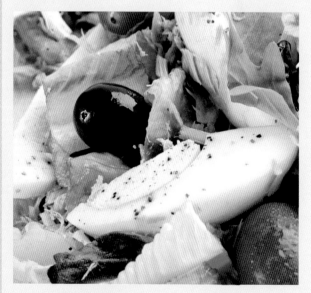

Chicken salad with sesame dressing

Chicken is high in protein and low in fat. It also provides B vitamins. Sesame oil rich in omega 3 oils and vitamin E. Add other vegetables, such as mushrooms or radishes, which work well with the dressing.

MAKES 4 SERVINGS

- 125 g (4 oz.) pack ready-washed salad leaves
- 1 cucumber, sliced diagonally
- A small handful of chopped fresh mint
- 4 skinless boneless chicken breasts

For dressing:

- 125 ml (4 fl oz.) rice vinegar
- 1 tbsp (15 ml.) Dijon mustard
- 2 tbsp (30 ml.) olive oil
- 2 tbsp (30 ml.) sesame oil
- 2 tsp (10 ml.) soy sauce
- 4 spring onions, chopped

1 *Make the dressing: whisk the vinegar and mustard in a bowl. Gradually whisk in both oils, then the soy sauce. Mix in the spring onions.*

2 *Place the chicken in a large glass baking dish. Pour half the dressing over and turn to coat. Cover and chill for at least 30 minutes.*

3 *Pre-heat the grill. Remove chicken from marinade and cook under the grill, about 4 minutes per side for the chicken. Slice the cooked chicken.*

4 *Combine the salad leaves, cucumbers and mint in large bowl. Pour enough dressing over salad to coat and toss gently. Transfer to large plate and spoon the chicken slices on top.*

Chickpea salad with walnuts

Chickpeas are an excellent source of fibre, protein and iron. Watercress is also rich in iron as well as vitamin C, beta-carotene and folate.

MAKES 4 SERVINGS

- 400 g (14 oz.) tin chickpeas, drained and rinsed
- 1 red onion, thinly sliced
- 1 red pepper, deseeded and sliced
- 100 g (3.5 oz.) of ready-washed watercress
- 85 g (3 oz.) walnuts, lightly toasted

Dressing:

- 3 tablespoons (45 ml.) extra virgin olive oil
- 2 tablespoons (30 ml.) balsamic vinegar
- 1 garlic clove, crushed
- 1 teaspoon (5 ml.) Dijon mustard

1 *In a large bowl, mix together the chickpeas, onion, pepper and olives.*

2 *Place the dressing ingredients in a screw-topped glass jar and shake until combined. Add half of the dressing to the chickpea salad and mix.*

3 *Toss the watercress with the remaining dressing. Transfer to a serving plate.*

4 *Spoon the chickpeas over the leaves then scatter over the toasted walnuts.*

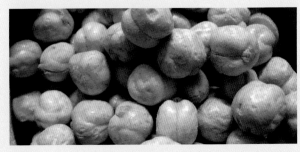

Chicken noodle salad

This salad provides a near-perfect balance of protein and carbohydrate, as well as plenty of fibre, vitamin C (from the mange tout and Chinese leaves) and vitamin A (from the carrots).

MAKES 4 SERVINGS

- 3 tbsp soy sauce
- 2 garlic cloves, crushed
- 1 tbsp olive or sesame oil
- 300 g (10 oz.) chicken fillet, cut into strips
- 350 g (12 oz.) noodles
- 400 g (14 oz.) mange tout
- 225 g (8 oz.) beansprouts
- 200 g (7 oz.) Chinese leaves or spring greens, chopped
- 225 g (8 oz.) carrots, grated
- Season with lemon juice

1 *Combine the soy sauce, garlic cloves and oil in a bowl. Add the chicken, stir to coat and leave to marinate in the fridge for 1 hour or longer.*
2 *Cook the noodles according to directions on the packet. Drain.*
3 *In a large bowl, combine the noodles, mange tout, bean sprouts, carrots and Chinese leaves.*
4 *Dry-fry the chicken in a nonstick pan until cooked through. Toss in the salad and season with the lemon juice.*

Rice salad with apricots and almonds

Wholegrain (brown) rice comprises the whole of the rice grain, including the surrounding bran layers, which contain the fibre, magnesium, phosphorus, thiamin (vitamin B1) and iron, which are necessary in our diet.

MAKES 4 SERVINGS

- 225 g (8 oz.) wholegrain (brown) rice
- 2 tbsp extra virgin olive oil
- 1 onion, peeled and chopped
- 2 cloves of garlic, crushed
- 60 g (2 oz.) flaked almonds
- 1 tbsp lemon juice
- 85 g (3 oz.) ready-to-eat dried apricots
- 2 tbsp chopped fresh coriander

1 *Bring a large pan of water to the boil. Stir in the rice. Cover and simmer for the time recommended on the packet. Drain. Alternatively, cook the rice in twice its own volume of water until the water has been absorbed.*
2 *Meanwhile, heat the olive oil in a pan, add the onion and garlic and cook over a moderate heat for 5 minutes until they are translucent.*
3 *Turn up the heat, add the almonds and cook for a few minutes longer, stirring often, until the onion and nuts are golden brown.*
4 *Add the onion mixture to the rice, along with the lemon juice, the apricots and coriander. Mix together then transfer to a serving dish.*

Hummus

Although hummus is widely available in supermarkets, it's worth making your own so you can reduce the salt and oil content. This tasty dip is delicious in sandwiches (made with non-wheat bread) or spread on rye crackers and rice cakes.

MAKES 4 SERVINGS

- 125 g (4 oz.) chickpeas, soaked overnight (or use a
- 400 g/ 14 oz. tin, drained and rinsed)
- 2 garlic cloves, crushed
- 2 tbsp olive oil
- 120 ml (4 fl oz.) tahini
- Juice of 1 lemon
- Pinch of paprika or cayenne pepper
- Freshly ground black pepper

1 *Drain then cook the chickpeas in plenty of water for approximately 60–90 minutes or according to directions on the packet. Drain, reserving the liquid.*
2 *Purée the cooked chickpeas with the remaining ingredients, with enough of the cooking liquid to make a creamy consistency.*
3 *Taste and add more black pepper or lemon juice if necessary.*
4 *Chill in the fridge for at least 2 hours before serving.*

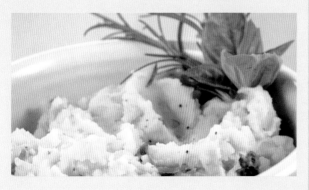

Guacamole (avocado dip)

Avocados are brimming with heart-healthy nutrients: monounsaturated oils, vitamin E, folic acid and potassium. This dip is easy to make and can be used as a sandwich spread, a dip for vegetable crudités or for spooning on salads.

MAKES 4 SERVINGS

- 2 ripe avocados
- 2 tbsp lemon or lime juice
- ½ small red onion, finely chopped
- 1 clove of garlic, crushed
- 2 medium tomatoes, skinned and chopped
- 2 tbsp fresh coriander, finely chopped
- Sea salt and freshly ground black pepper

- *To serve:* cayenne pepper and extra virgin olive oil

1 *Halve the avocados and scoop out the flesh. Mash the avocado flesh with the lemon or lime juice.*
2 *Add the remaining ingredients, mixing well. Alternatively, you may process the ingredients in a food processor to a coarse purée.*
3 *Check the seasoning, adding a little more black pepper or lemon juice if necessary. Chill.*
4 *Before serving sprinkle with a little cayenne pepper and drizzle with olive oil.*

Salad dressings

Try any of the following for a super quick dressing:

- A drizzle of balsamic vinegar or flavoured vinegar (e.g. raspberry, rosemary, basil, garlic)
- A squeeze of lime juice or lemon juice
- Low fat fromage frais mixed with a little mint sauce or wholegrain mustard
- Plain yogurt mixed with lemon juice
- Equal quantities of pesto and yogurt
- Low fat salad dressing or mayonnaise mixed with curry powder

Garlic and herb dressing

- 60 ml (2 fl oz.) red wine vinegar
- 2 tbsp orange juice
- 1 tbsp extra virgin olive oil
- 1 crushed garlic clove
- 1 tbsp chopped fresh parsley
- 1 tbsp chopped fresh tarragon

Place the ingredients in a screw top jar and shake well to combine.

Honey and mustard dressing

- 5 tbsp extra-virgin olive oil
- 2 tbsp cider vinegar
- ½ tsp Dijon mustard
- 1 level tsp clear honey
- ½ clove of garlic

Place all of the ingredients in a bottle or screw-top jar and shake well.

Tangy yogurt dressing

- 60 ml (2 fl oz) plain yogurt
- 2 tbsp orange juice
- 1 tbsp honey
- 2 tsp Dijon mustard
- ¼ tsp ground ginger

Mix all the ingredients together thoroughly in a small bowl.

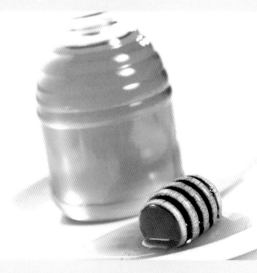

PASTA, RICE AND OTHER GRAINS

Athletes hot pasta with vegetables

This basic pasta recipe takes less than 15 minutes to prepare making it ideal for quick nutritious suppers. Simply add whatever fresh or frozen vegetables you have handy to the pasta pot. Any leftovers are also good served cold as a salad.

MAKES 4 SERVINGS

- 350 g (12 oz.) dried pasta of your choice
- 2 tbsp olive oil
- 1 onion, chopped
- 2 garlic cloves, crushed
- 400 g (14 oz.) tin chopped tomatoes
- 2 tbsp tomato purée
- 2 or more vegetables from list below*
- 1 tbsp chopped fresh basil or 1 tsp dried basil
- 25 g (1 oz.) Parmesan, grated
- *Vegetables for the sauce:*
- asparagus, chopped into 4 cm (1.5 in.) lengths; sliced courgettes; chopped red, green or yellow peppers; small broccoli florets; mange tout; chopped aubergine; sliced mushrooms; peas; French beans, chopped into 4 cm (1.5 in.) lengths.

1 *Cook the pasta in plenty of boiling water according to the directions on the packet.*
2 *Meanwhile, heat the oil in a large pan. Add the onions and garlic and cook over a moderate heat for 5 minutes. Add the tomatoes, tomato purée, prepared vegetables and basil.*
3 *Cook for 4 minutes, or until the vegetables are tender but still firm.*
4 *Combine the sauce with the pasta, and then scatter over the Parmesan.*

Vegetarian Bolognese pasta sauce

Packed with protein, fibre and iron, this delicious pasta sauce goes well with spaghetti and tagliatelle.

MAKES 4 SERVINGS

- 1 tbsp olive oil
- 1 onion, chopped
- 2 carrots, finely chopped
- 1 large courgette, finely chopped
- 1 400 g (14 oz.) tin chopped tomatoes
- 1 420 g (15 oz.) tin brown or green lentils, or 125 g (4 oz.) dried lentils, soaked and cooked
- 1 tsp mixed herbs
- 1 tbsp parmesan, grated

1 *Heat the oil in a large frying pan. Add the vegetables; cook stirring often until softened (approximately 5 minutes).*
2 *Add the tomatoes, lentils and herbs. Cook until the sauce thickens slightly.*
3 *Stir in the cheese and heat through.*

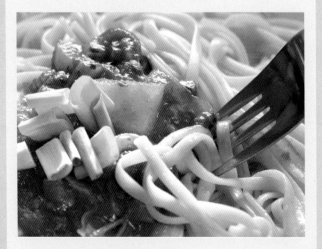

Turkey Bolognese pasta sauce

Turkey mince has a lower fat content than ordinary beef mince. It is also high in protein, B vitamins and iron. The vegetables add extra fibre and vitamins.

MAKES 4 SERVINGS

- 1 tsp olive oil
- 350 g (12 oz.) turkey mince
- 1 onion, chopped
- 3 celery stalks, chopped
- 2 carrots, chopped
- 1 400 g (14 oz.) tin chopped tomatoes
- 2 tbsp tomato purée
- 1 tsp mixed herbs
- Salt and pepper

1 *In a large nonstick frying pan, heat the oil. Add the turkey mince and cook, stirring for approximately 4–5 minutes until no longer pink.*
2 *Add the vegetables. Cook for 3–5 minutes until just tender.*
3 *Stir in the chopped tomatoes, tomato purée, herbs and seasoning to taste.*
4 *Heat through.*

Tomato and tuna pasta sauce

This simple pasta sauce can be prepared in just 10 minutes. It is bursting with antioxidant nutrients (from the tomatoes) and protein (from the tuna) and contains far less salt than ready-bought versions.

MAKES 4 SERVINGS

- 1 onion, chopped
- 1 garlic clove, crushed
- 1 400 g (14 oz.) tin chopped tomatoes
- 1 tbsp tomato purée
- 125 g (4 oz.) vegetable of choice
  (e.g. mushrooms, courgettes)
- 1 200 g (7 oz.) tin tuna in water or brine,
  drained and flaked
- 1 tsp dried basil

1 *Place the onion, garlic and tomatoes in a large nonstick frying pan and cook for 4–5 minutes until onion is soft.*
2 *Stir in the tomato purée and vegetables and cook for 5 minutes.*
3 *Add the tuna and basil and heat through.*

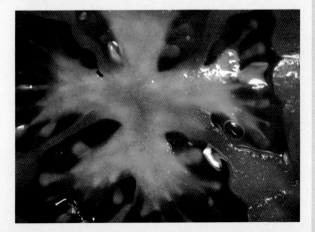

Cheese sauce

This recipe has a lower fat content than the traditional version as it omits the butter and uses semi-skimmed milk instead of full fat milk. I prefer using cornflour instead of ordinary flour, as you need use only half as much and, as it dissolves in cold liquid, it greatly reduces the risk of getting a lumpy sauce.

MAKES 4 SERVINGS

- 600 ml (1 pt.) semi-skimmed milk
- 2 level tbsp cornflour
- ½ tsp Dijon mustard
- 85 g (3 oz.) extra mature Cheddar cheese, grated
- Freshly ground black pepper

1 *Blend the cornflour with a little of the milk in a jug. Gradually add the remainder of the milk, stirring to ensure a smooth sauce.*
2 *Pour into a saucepan and heat, stirring constantly until the sauce just reaches the boil and has thickened.*
3 *Remove from the heat, stir in the mustard, cheese and freshly ground black pepper to taste. Serve straight away to prevent a skin forming over the surface.*

Ham and mushroom sauce

Try substituting 4 boneless chicken breasts (approx. 85 g/ 3 oz. each), sliced into 1 cm (½ in.) strips for the ham.

MAKES 4 SERVINGS

- 1 tsp oil
- 4 slices (125 g/4.4 oz.) ham (preferably reduced salt), chopped
- 225 g (8 oz.) small mushrooms, halved
- 2 tbsp cornflour
- 600 ml (1 pt.) semi-skimmed milk
- 1 tsp dried oregano or basil
- Freshly ground black pepper

1 *Heat the oil in a large frying pan. Cook the ham and mushrooms for 4–5 minutes.*
2 *Stir in the cornflour together with a little milk. Gradually add the rest of the milk, stirring continuously.*
3 *Heat until it just reaches boiling point. Remove from the heat and stir in the herbs and pepper.*

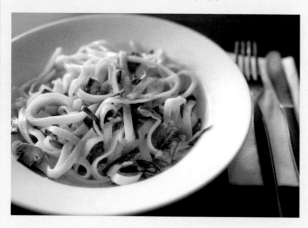

Macaroni cheese with vegetables

Not only is this version of the classic dish lower in fat, it also includes extra vegetables to boost the fibre and vitamin content.

MAKES 4 SERVINGS

- 1 tsp olive oil
- 1 large onion, sliced
- 250 g (8 oz.) sliced vegetables of your choice (e.g. mushrooms, peppers, tomatoes, courgettes)
- 2 tbsp low fat spread
- 2 tbsp cornflour
- 600 ml (1 pt.) skimmed milk
- 60 g (2 oz.) mature (strong) Cheddar cheese
- 350 g (12 oz.) macaroni

1 *In a nonstick pan, sauté the vegetables in the olive oil over a high heat until browned.*
2 *Whisk together the low fat spread, cornflour and milk in a saucepan over a medium heat until thickened. Stir in the cheese.*
3 *Meanwhile boil the macaroni for about 10 minutes. Drain.*
4 *In a large baking dish, layer the half macaroni, vegetables and sauce. Repeat, finishing with a layer of sauce.*
5 *Bake in an oven at 180°C/350°F/Gas mark 4 until hot and bubbly, for approximately 20 minutes.*

Pasta and tuna bake

High in carbohydrate, protein and calcium, this dish is easy to prepare and can be varied according to what vegetables you have to hand. Try adding sliced peppers, courgettes or tomatoes.

MAKES 4 SERVINGS

- 2 tsp olive oil
- 1 onion, sliced
- 3 sticks of celery, chopped
- 125 g (4 oz.) mushrooms, sliced
- 350 g (12 oz.) dry weight pasta shells
- 3 tbsp fresh parsley, chopped
- 1 200 g (7 oz.) tin tuna in water, drained

White Sauce:
- 1 tbsp low fat spread
- 1 tbsp cornflour
- 450 ml (¾ pt.) skimmed milk

1 *In a nonstick frying pan, sauté the vegetables in the olive oil.*
2 *Prepare the white sauce by whisking all the sauce ingredients in a saucepan over a medium heat until thickened.*
3 *Meanwhile, cook the pasta according to the packet directions. Drain.*
4 *Spoon layers of the vegetables, pasta, tuna and white sauce in to a baking dish, sprinkling parsley between each layer and finishing with a layer of the sauce.*
5 *Bake at 180 °C/375 °F/Gas mark 5 for 20 minutes. Alternatively cook in the microwave for 6 minutes.*

Lasagne

This recipe for lasagne has a lower fat content than the traditional version as it uses lean meat and low-fat cheese instead of cheese sauce.

MAKES 4 SERVINGS

- 1 onion, chopped
- 2 courgettes, sliced
- 225 g (8 oz.) extra lean beef mince (or turkey mince)
- 1 400 g (14 oz.) tin chopped tomatoes
- 3 tbsp tomato purée
- 1 tsp basil or oregano
- Salt and pepper to taste
- 12 sheets lasagne (no pre-cook variety)
- 350 g (12 oz.) cottage cheese
- 85 g (3 oz.) reduced fat mozzarella
- You may add other vegetables e.g. mushrooms, peppers, spinach, to the mince mixture instead of the courgettes.

1 *Heat a large nonstick frying pan. Cook the onion, courgette and mince, stirring frequently, for 5–6 minutes until the mince is no longer pink. Drain off any fat.*
2 *Add the tomatoes, tomato purée, and herbs. Season with salt and pepper to taste.*
3 *Place four sheets of lasagne at the bottom of an oiled baking dish. Spoon over one-third of the meat mixture and one-third of the cottage cheese. Repeat the layers, finishing with a layer of cottage cheese.*
4 *Cover with very thin slices of mozzarella.*
5 *Bake at 180 °C/350 °F/Gas mark 4 for 30 minutes.*

Pasta with chicken and mushrooms

This simple one-pot pasta meal provides a good balance of protein, complex carbohydrate, vitamins and minerals. Add tinned beans, such as red kidney beans, for extra fibre and iron.

MAKES 4 SERVINGS

- 4 chicken drumsticks or thighs, skinned
- 1 tbsp olive oil
- 1 onion, sliced
- 2 green or red peppers, sliced
- 225 g (8 oz.) mushrooms, sliced
- 450 ml (16 fl oz.) passata (sieved tomatoes)
- 350 g (12 oz.) small pasta shapes
- 285 ml (½ pt.) stock or water

1 Sauté the chicken drumsticks in the oil over a high heat until it is browned. Remove from pan and set aside on a plate.
2 Add the onions, peppers and mushrooms to the pan and cook for 5–10 minutes.
3 Add the passata, chicken, pasta and stock or water. Bring to the boil and simmer until the pasta is tender and the chicken cooked through, about 10 minutes.
4 Accompany with warm French bread.

Vegetable paella

This is a vegetarian version of the classic Spanish paella that uses vegetables instead of the fish. The peas add protein to the dish.

MAKES 4 SERVINGS

- 2 tablespoons oil
- 1 onion, chopped
- 2 garlic cloves, crushed
- 4 celery sticks, chopped
- 1 red, yellow and green pepper, sliced
- 1 tsp paprika
- 350 g (12 oz.) rice
- 1 400 g (14 oz.) tin chopped tomatoes
- 900 ml (1.5 pt.) vegetable stock (or water plus 2 vegetable stock cubes)
- 225 g (8 oz.) frozen peas
- Salt and pepper to taste
- *Optional:*
- 2 tbsp chopped parsley
- 60 g (2 oz.) black olives

1 Heat the oil in a large pan and sauté the onion, garlic, celery and peppers for 5 minutes.
2 Add the paprika and rice and stir for another 2–3 minutes.
3 Add the tomatoes and stock, bring to the boil then simmer for 15 –20 minutes until the liquid has been absorbed.
4 Add the peas, season to taste and heat through for a few more minutes.
5 Stir in the optional ingredients.

Lemon rice with chickpeas and spinach

Basmati rice has a lower GI than ordinary rice. In this dish, it is combined with chickpeas, which also has a low GI. Eat this 3–4 hours before an endurance workout for sustained energy.

MAKES 4 SERVINGS

- 225 g (8 oz.) basmati rice
- Zest of 1 lemon
- 1 × 425 g (15 oz.) tin chickpeas, drained
- 125 g (4 oz) baby spinach leaves
- 60 g (2 oz) black olives (pitted)
- A little low-sodium salt and freshly ground black pepper

1 *Put the basmati rice, lemon zest and 400 ml (14 fl oz.) water in a large saucepan. Bring to the boil. Cover, reduce the heat and simmer for 15 minutes.*
2 *Add the chickpeas and continue cooking over a gentle heat for a further 5–10 minutes until the liquid has been absorbed and the rice is cooked. Add the spinach and let stand for another couple of minutes.*
3 *Stir in the olives, season with the low sodium salt and pepper and serve.*

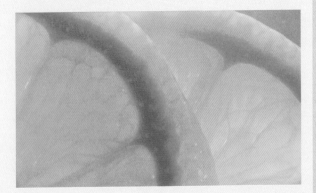

Chicken and mixed pepper risotto

This is a cheat's risotto as everything is cooked together to save time. However, the result is tasty and the peppers provide an excellent source of vitamin C and beta-carotene.

MAKES 4 SERVINGS

- 2 l (3.5 pt.) chicken or vegetable stock
- 350 g (12 oz.) white rice
- 2 peppers, preferably one red, one yellow, cut into thin strips
- 125 g (4 oz.) cooked chicken, chopped
- 25 g (1 oz.) parmesan, grated
- Handful of fresh chives or parsley, if available

1 *Place the stock, rice and peppers in a large saucepan.*
2 *Bring to the boil and simmer for 12–15 minutes until the rice is tender and the liquid has been absorbed.*
3 *Add the chicken and half the parmesan. Heat through for a few minutes.*
4 *Serve topped with remaining parmesan and herbs.*

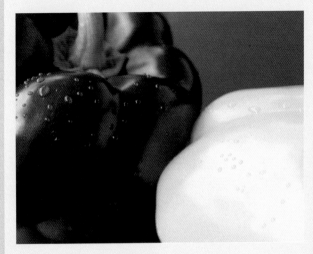

Fruit and nut pilaf

Vary this basic recipe with any seasonal vegetables you have to hand. Whichever ones you use, this dish provides an excellent source of slow-release energy together with fibre, vitamins and minerals from the vegetables. The nuts supply extra protein and healthy fats.

MAKES 4 SERVINGS

- 2 tbsp olive oil
- 1 onion, chopped
- 2 garlic cloves, crushed
- 4 celery sticks, chopped
- 1 red, yellow and green pepper, sliced
- 300 g (10 oz.) brown rice
- 900 ml (1.5 pt.) vegetable stock
- 100 g (3.5 oz.) mixture of nuts and raisins (e.g. almonds, cashews, walnuts)
- Handful of fresh parsley, chopped
- Salt and freshly ground pepper to taste

1 *Heat the oil in a large saucepan and sauté the onion over a gentle heat for 2 minutes. Add the garlic, celery and peppers and continue cooking for 3–4 minutes.*
2 *Stir in the brown rice and cook, while continuously stirring, for a further 2 minutes until the grains become translucent.*
3 *Add the vegetable stock, bring to the boil then simmer for 20–25 minutes until the liquid has been absorbed and the rice is cooked.*
4 *Stir in the fruit and nut mixture, and the parsley, then season to taste with the salt and freshly ground black pepper.*

Butternut squash risotto

Butternut squash is super-rich in beta-carotene, which has powerful antioxidant properties, helping protect against heart disease and cancer. It also benefits the skin and can be converted into vitamin A in the body.

MAKES 4 SERVINGS

- 3 tbsp (45 ml.) extra virgin olive oil
- 1 large onion, chopped
- 1 tsp ground cumin
- 1 tsp ground coriander
- 300 g (10 oz.) Arborio (risotto) rice
- 1 litre (1¾ pt.) hot vegetable stock
- 350 g (12 oz.) butternut squash, peeled, deseeded and cut into 12 mm (0.5 in.) pieces
- 1 medium courgette, diced
- 125 g (4 oz.) fresh or frozen peas
- 1 tbsp (15 ml.) fresh chopped parsley
- Sea salt and black pepper
- 30 g (1 oz.) flaked toasted almonds

1 *Heat the olive oil in a large pan. Add the onion and cook for 2 minutes until translucent. Stir in the spices and continue cooking for a further minute.*
2 *Add the rice and stir until the grains are coated with the oil. Add the hot vegetable stock one ladle at a time; stir and simmer for approximately 10 minutes.*
3 *Add the butternut squash and courgette; continue cooking for a further 5 minutes.*
4 *Add the peas and continue cooking for a further 5 minutes until all the liquid has been absorbed and the rice is tender but firm in the centre. Perfect risotto is creamy but not solid, and the rice should still have a little bite.*
5 *Stir in the parsley and season to taste. Scatter over the almonds and serve immediately.*

Beans 'n' rice

This is a vegetarian adaptation of the traditional West Indian dish. The combination of beans and rice increases the overall protein value of the dish. It can be made as spicy, hot or mild as you wish.

MAKES 4 SERVINGS

- 1 tbsp oil
- 1 onion, chopped
- 1 green chilli, seeded and finely chopped
- 350 g (12 oz.) rice
- 900 ml (1½ pt.) vegetable stock (or water plus 2 vegetable stock cubes)
- 2 large tomatoes, sliced
- 1 420 g (15 oz.) tin black, white or red beans *
- 60 g (2 oz) creamed coconut
- 2 tbsp fresh chopped coriander or parsley

* Either red kidney beans; aduki; cannelini; haricot or black beans.

1 *Heat the oil in a pan and fry the onion for approximately 5 minutes. Add the chilli and rice and fry for a further 2 minutes.*
2 *Add the stock and tomato, bring to the boil and simmer for 10 minutes.*
3 *Add the beans and a little extra water if the mixture looks dry. Cover and cook for a further 5 minutes until the rice is cooked.*
4 *Stir in the coconut until it is melted and then stir in the coriander or parsley.*

Noodles with salmon in foil

This complete meal comes in a neat packet; you just pop in the ingredients and put it in the oven. Meanwhile all the flavours blend together in the oven.

MAKES 1 SERVING

- 85 g (3 oz.) egg noodles, cooked according to directions on packet
- 1 carrot, thinly sliced
- 2 spring onions, sliced
- 4 mushrooms
- 1 salmon steak (about 175 g/6 oz.)
- Fresh chopped parsley

1 *Place the noodles onto the centre of a piece of oiled foil approx 50 × 30 cm (20 × 12 in.).*
2 *Lay the vegetables and salmon on top. Sprinkle with salt and parsley.*
   Fold the foil over to enclose the salmon and seal the edges. Place on a baking tray.
3 *Bake at 180 °C/350 °F/Gas mark 4 for 15 minutes.*
4 *Turn onto a plate to serve.*

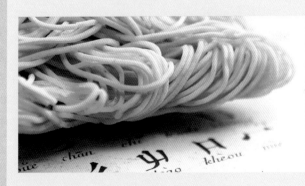

Couscous with roasted vegetables, nuts and fruit

MAKES 4 SERVINGS

- ½ red pepper
- ½ yellow pepper
- 200 g (7 oz.) cherry tomatoes, halved
- 1 courgette, sliced
- 2 tbsp (30 ml.) extra virgin olive oil
- 250 g (9 oz.) couscous
- 400 ml (⅔ pt.) hot vegetable stock or water
- 100 g (3.5 oz.) packet fruit and nut mix
- A small handful of fresh coriander, chopped
- A little low-sodium salt and freshly ground black pepper

1 *Pre-heat the oven to 200°C/400°F/Gas mark 6.*
2 *Remove the seeds from the peppers and cut them into wide strips. Place in a large roasting tin with the courgette slices and cherry tomatoes. Drizzle over the olive oil and toss lightly so that the vegetables are well coated in the oil.*
3 *Roast in the oven for approximately 30 minutes until the peppers are slightly charred on the outside and tender in the middle. Allow to cool, then roughly chop the peppers.*
4 *Put the couscous in a large bowl and cover with the hot stock or water. Stir briefly, cover and allow to stand for 5 minutes until the stock has been absorbed. Fluff up with a fork.*
5 *Add the roasted vegetables, fruit and nut mix and coriander. Season to taste with the low sodium salt and black pepper. Serve.*

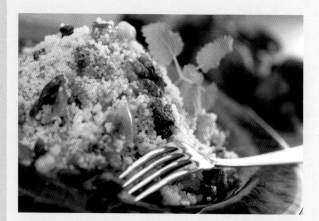

Millet pilaf with almonds

Millet has a delicate slightly nutty flavour. It has a higher protein and iron content than most other grains. This dish is also a good source of vitamins A and E.

MAKES 4 SERVINGS

- 1 tbsp oil
- 1 large onion, chopped
- 2 carrots, diced
- 1 garlic clove, crushed
- 350 g (12 oz.) millet
- 900 ml (1½ pt.) water
- Season with salt and freshly ground black pepper
- 60 g (2 oz.) raisins
- 60 g (2 oz.) toasted flaked almonds

1 *Heat the oil in a saucepan and cook the onion for 5 minutes. Add the carrots and garlic and cook for a further 5 minutes.*
2 *Add the millet and water and season to taste with the salt and pepper. Bring to the boil, cover and simmer for 15–20 minutes until the water has been absorbed.*
3 *Stir in the raisins and almonds.*

MAIN MEALS

Fish and bean cassoulet

This nutritious dish is packed with protein, vitamins and fibre. Substitute other types of white fish if you wish. Try adding courgettes, red peppers, aubergine or butternut squash.

MAKES 4 SERVINGS

- 750 g (1.5 lb.) haddock steaks
- 1 l (1.75 pt.) stock or water
- 1 bay leaf
- 1 tbsp oil
- 1 onion, chopped
- 2 celery sticks, chopped
- 2 carrots, chopped
- 4 tbsp white wine or water
- 400 g (14 oz.) can haricot beans, drained
- 1 tsp mixed herbs
- 4 tomatoes, chopped
- 4 tbsp fresh breadcrumbs
- 2 tbsp fresh chopped parsley

1 *Cook the fish in the stock or water with the bay leaf for approximately 10–15 minutes. Drain, reserving 1 pint of the liquid.*
2 *Flake the fish, removing any bones.*
3 *Heat the oil in a pan and fry the vegetables for approximately 5 minutes.*
4 *Pour in the reserved fish liquid, wine or extra water, beans and herbs and cook for approximately 10 minutes until the liquid has been reduced.*
5 *Add the cooked fish and tomatoes. Check the seasoning and transfer into a shallow baking dish.*
6 *Mix the breadcrumbs and parsley together and scatter over the top.*
7 *Bake at 190°C/375°F/Gas mark 5 for 30–35 minutes until the top is crisp and golden.*

Stir-fried chicken with broccoli

Chicken provides protein and B vitamins. Broccoli is rich in sulphoramine, a powerful antioxidant that fights cancer, as well as vitamin C and folate.

MAKES 4 SERVINGS

- 2 tbsp extra virgin olive oil
- 300 g (10 oz.) chicken breasts cut into thin strips
- 1 tbsp light (low sodium) soy sauce
- 1 onion, thinly sliced
- 2.5 cm (1 in.) piece fresh ginger, peeled and finely chopped
- 225 g (8 oz.) broccoli florets
- 1 tsp cornflour blended with 1 tbsp water
- A handful of fresh chives, chopped

1 *Heat the olive oil in a wok, add the chicken and stir-fry for 2–3 minutes until the chicken is lightly browned. Remove from the wok, place on a plate and keep warm.*
2 *Add the onion and ginger and stir-fry for 1 minute. Add the broccoli then return the chicken to the wok.*
3 *Pour over the cornflour mixture, stirring continuously, until the mixture thickens.*
4 *Serve with cooked rice or noodles.*

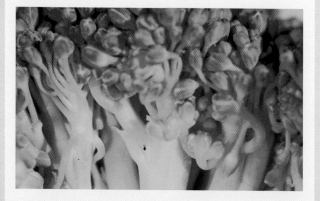

Lean meat burgers

These homemade meat burgers are made with lean mince and cooked without extra oil. This means they are low in fat – and at least you know exactly what's in them!

MAKES 4 BURGERS

- 350 g (12 oz.) extra lean minced meat (beef, turkey, pork)
- 60 g (2 oz.) dried breadcrumbs
- 3 tbsp water
- 1 small onion, chopped
- 2 tbsp fresh sage or parsley, chopped (or 1 tbsp dried)
- Freshly ground black pepper

1 *Place the minced meat, breadcrumbs, water, onion, herbs and pepper in a bowl. Mix well to combine.*
2 *Divide the mixture into four balls and flatten into burgers.*
3 *Dry fry in a hot nonstick pan for 3–4 minutes each side. Alternatively, place the burgers on a baking sheet and cook in the oven at 200 °C/400 °F/Gas mark 6 for 10–15 minutes depending on the size of the burgers. Test by inserting a skewer into the middle of a burger – there should be no trace of pink in the meat and the juices should run clear.*

Chicken burgers

These are a healthy alternative to beef burgers due to their lower fat content.

MAKES 4 BURGERS

- 1 onion, finely chopped
- 1 stick celery, finely chopped
- 1 clove garlic, crushed
- 2 tbsp olive oil
- 2 chicken breasts, skinless and boneless
- 2 tbsp fresh parsley, chopped (or 1 tbsp dried parsley)
- 60 g (2 oz.) fresh breadcrumbs
- Salt and freshly ground black pepper
- 1 egg yolk
- Flour for coating

1 *Sauté the onion, celery and garlic in the olive oil for 5 minutes. Meanwhile mince or finely chop the chicken in a food processor.*
2 *Combine the onion mixture, chicken, parsley and breadcrumbs in a bowl. Season with salt and pepper and bind the mixture together with the egg yolk.*
3 *Form into four burgers and roll in a little flour.*
4 *Dry-fry in a nonstick pan over a medium heat until golden, turning halfway through (approximately 5–6 minutes each side).*

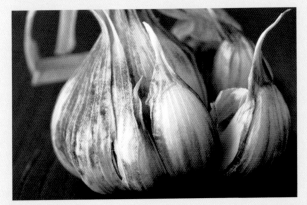

Mackerel with fresh coriander & chilli dressing

This recipe is ultra quick to make and full of healthy omega 3 fatty acids.

MAKES 4 SERVINGS

- 4 mackerel each weighing about 350 g (12 oz.), gutted
- Oil for brushing
- Salt and freshly ground black pepper

For the dressing:
- 2 shallots, very finely chopped
- 2 plump garlic cloves, crushed
- 1 fresh red chilli, deseeded and chopped
- 6 tbsp extra virgin olive oil
- Juice of 1 lemon
- 4 tbsp fresh coriander, chopped

1 *Put all the dressing ingredients into a small bowl and mix well. Put aside until ready to use.*
2 *Make three to four deep slashes on each side of the mackerel. Brush with a little oil and season inside and out.*
3 *Grill on a barbecue or under a hot conventional grill for 8–10 minutes, turning once halfway through cooking.*
4 *Put the fish on a warm dish, pour over the dressing and leave for 5 minutes to let it infuse. Serve with couscous.*

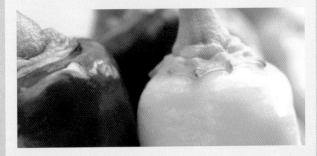

Chicken with courgettes

Infusing chicken thighs in this tasty citrus marinade helps reduce the formation of potentially carcinogenic chemicals during barbecuing.

MAKES 4 SERVINGS

- Zest and juice of 1 lemon
- 1 tbsp olive oil
- ½ tsp salt
- ¼ tsp coarsely ground black pepper
- 4 medium skinless, boneless chicken thighs
- 4 medium courgettes, each cut lengthwise into 4 wedges
- Small handful of fresh chives, snipped
- Grilled lemon slices for garnish

1 *In a medium bowl, whisk together the lemon zest and juice, oil, salt, and pepper. Transfer 2 tablespoons to a cup.*

2 *Add the chicken thighs to the bowl of marinade. Cover and leave to stand for 15 minutes at room temperature or 30 minutes in the refrigerator.*

3 *Discard chicken marinade. Place chicken and courgettes on a hot barbecue grill rack. Cover grill and cook for 10–12 minutes or until juices run clear when thickest part of thigh is pierced with tip of knife and the courgettes are tender and lightly browned. Turn chicken and vegetables over once and remove pieces as they are done.*

4 *To serve, toss the courgettes with reserved lemon juice marinade, then combine with chicken and sprinkle with chives. Garnish with grilled lemon slices.*

Roasted winter vegetables with oat-crusted salmon

The lightly toasted oat crust adds extra flavour and nutrients. Salmon is a concentrated source of omega-3 fatty acids, which help reduce the risk of heart attacks and stroke, as well as benefiting the skin, reducing the appearance of wrinkles and helping to control blood pressure.

MAKES 4 SERVINGS

- 2 × 300 g (10 oz.) salmon fillets, skinned
- 4 carrots, peeled and halved
- 2 parsnips, peeled and cut in to quarters
- 2 red onions, cut into wedges
- 2 leeks, sliced into 2.5 cm (1 in.) pieces
- ½ butternut squash, peeled and thickly sliced
- 1 garlic clove, crushed
- A few sprigs of fresh or dried rosemary
- A little low-sodium salt and freshly ground black pepper
- 1–2 tbsp olive oil
- 4 tbsp porridge oats
- 2 tbsp sesame seeds
- Lemon wedges to serve

1 *Pre-heat the oven to 200°C/400°F/Gas mark 6.*

2 *Prepare the vegetables and place in a large roasting tin. Scatter over the crushed garlic, rosemary, low sodium salt and black pepper. Drizzle over the oil. Roast in the oven for 30–40 minutes until tender.*

3 *Meanwhile, cut the salmon in half. Mix the porridge oats, sesame seeds, low sodium salt and black pepper. Dip each salmon portion in the oat mixture, coating the fish evenly.*

4 *Brush a nonstick frying pan or griddle with a little olive oil, heat then add the salmon. Cook over a moderate heat for 3 minutes on each side, covering with a lid. The salmon should be light brown and crispy on the outside.*

5 *Divide the roasted vegetables, place a salmon fillet on top and serve with the lemon wedges.*

175

Lamb kebabs with caper dip

Lamb is an excellent source of easily absorbed iron, as well as zinc, protein and B vitamins. Choose lean steaks and trim off any visible fat – this reduces the fat content to around 9 g (0.3 oz.) per 100 g (3.5 oz.).

MAKES 4 KEBABS

- 450 g (1 lb.) lean lamb leg steaks
- 2 red onions, cut into chunks
- 60 g (2 oz.) butter
- A few sprigs of fresh rosemary

For the caper dip:
- 2 tbsp capers, drained and rinsed
- 3 pickled gherkins, chopped
- 1 tbsp wholegrain mustard
- 1 tbsp white wine vinegar
- 1 tbsp fresh mint, chopped
- 1 tbsp fresh parsley, chopped
- 2 tbsp mayonnaise

1 *Cut the lamb leg steaks into 2.5 cm (1 in.) cubes and thread onto skewers with the red onion chunks.*
2 *Melt and add the fresh rosemary leaves, brush over the skewers and cook under a preheated grill for 12–15 minutes, turning occasionally.*
3 *Meanwhile make the caper dip: in a bowl mix together the capers, pickled gherkins, wholegrain mustard, white wine vinegar, fresh mint, fresh parsley, and mayonnaise.*
4 *Serve the kebabs with the caper dip on a bed of healthy brown rice, and a large mixed leaf salad.*

Chicken casserole with lentils and leeks

Chicken is a low fat source of protein as well as B vitamins, iron and zinc. In this healthy casserole, it is slow-cooked with Puy lentils, which provide a good balance of protein and complex carbohydrates as well as soluble fibre, iron, B vitamins, zinc and magnesium, and leeks, which are a great natural diuretic.

MAKES 4 SERVINGS

- 2 tbsp extra virgin olive oil
- 4 chicken breasts
- 2 leeks, trimmed and thickly sliced
- 1 onion, sliced
- 2 large carrots, peeled and sliced
- 4 sage leaves, roughly chopped
- 125 g (4 oz.) Puy lentils
- 500 ml (16 fl oz.) chicken stock
- A little low-sodium salt and freshly ground black pepper, to taste
- 2 tbsp chopped fresh parsley

1 *Heat the oven to 190 °C/375 °F/Gas mark 5.*
2 *Heat the oil in a flameproof casserole dish on top of the stove and brown the chicken.*
3 *Add the leeks, onions and carrots and continue cooking for a few minutes.*
4 *Add the sage, lentils and stock and bring to the boil. Season with low sodium salt and black pepper.*
5 *Cover and simmer in the oven for 1 hour or until the chicken is very tender, stirring halfway through cooking.*
6 *Stir in the parsley just before serving.*

Pan-fried salmon with vegetable rice and rocket

Salmon is rich in heart-healthy omega-3 oils as well as protein and vitamin E. This dish also provides complex carbohydrates, vitamin C, beta-carotene, fibre and iron.

MAKES 4 SERVINGS

- 1 tbsp olive oil
- 1 onion, chopped
- 1 garlic clove, crushed
- 2 courgettes, diced
- 1 red or yellow pepper, chopped
- 225 g (8 oz.) brown basmati rice
- 800 ml (1.5 pt.) vegetable stock
- 125 g (4 oz.) frozen peas
- A little salt (or low sodium salt) and freshly ground black pepper to taste
- 150 g (5 oz.) salmon fillet
- A handful of rocket

1 Heat the oil in a large pan and sauté the onion, garlic, courgettes and peppers for 5 minutes.
2 Add the rice and stir over the heat for a further 2–3 minutes.
3 Add the stock, bring to the boil, then reduce the heat and simmer for 25–30 minutes until the liquid has been absorbed.
4 Add the peas during the final 3 minutes of cooking. Season to taste.
5 Brush each salmon fillet with a little olive oil. Heat a nonstick pan until hot. Add the salmon fillets and fry for 4–5 minutes, turn over and cook the other side for 3 minutes. Remove from heat.
6 Divide the rice mixture onto four plates, scatter over the rocket. Place a salmon fillet on top and serve immediately.

Stir-fry Indonesian prawns in peanut sauce

MAKES 4 SERVINGS

- 225 g (8 oz.) green beans, cut in half
- 450 g (1 lb.) large peeled prawns
- 85 g (3 oz.) chunky peanut butter
- 150 ml (¼ pt.) unsweetened canned coconut milk
- 1 tbsp soy sauce
- 2 tsp curry powder
- A few spring onions, chopped

1 Place a wok over a high heat. Add the green beans and prawns and stir-fry for 3 minutes.
2 In a small bowl, whisk together the peanut butter, coconut milk, soy sauce, curry powder and 175 ml (6 fl oz.) water. Pour over the beans and prawns.
3 Add the spring onions. Stir and cook for a few minutes until warmed through and the sauce has thickened.
4 Serve with noodles or rice.

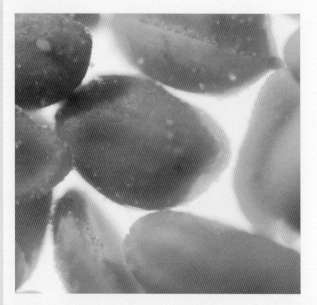

VEGETARIAN MAIN MEALS

Dahl with sweet potatoes

Red lentils are an excellent source of protein, complex carbohydrates, fibre, iron, zinc and B vitamins. They are low GI, perfect for pre-workout or post-workout meals. Sweet potatoes provide beta-carotene and vitamin C.

MAKES 4 SERVINGS

- 2 onions, chopped
- 2 tbsp rapeseed oil
- 2 garlic cloves, crushed
- 1 tsp ground cumin
- 2 tsp ground coriander
- 1 tsp turmeric
- 175 g (6 oz.) red lentils
- 750 ml (1¼ pt.) vegetable stock
- 1 sweet potato, peeled and diced
- 1 tbsp lemon juice
- A little low-sodium salt
- A small handful of fresh coriander, finely chopped

1 *Heat the oil in a heavy-based pan and sauté the onions for 5 minutes. Add the garlic and spices and continue cooking for 1 minute while stirring continuously.*

2 *Add the lentils, stock and sweet potatoes. Bring to the boil. Cover and simmer for approximately 20 minutes.*

3 *Add the lemon juice and low-sodium salt. Finally, stir in the fresh coriander.*

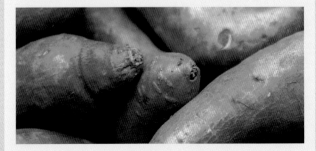

VEGETARIAN MAIN MEALS

Bean lasagne

This protein-packed lasagne is tasty enough to convert the most sceptical non-vegetarian. The beans provide complex carbs as well as fibre, iron, zinc and B vitamins. The cheeses supply bone-strengthening calcium.

MAKES 4 SERVINGS

- 1 onion, chopped
- 2 tsp olive oil
- 1 tsp each cumin and coriander
- 2 tins (2 × 420 g/15 oz.) mixed beans (or any variety of your choice), drained
- 1 tin (400 g/ 14 oz.) chopped tomatoes
- 12 sheets no pre-cook lasagne
- 350 g (12 oz.) cottage cheese
- 40 g (1½ oz.) reduced fat mozzarella, grated

1 *Pre-heat the oven to at 180 °C/350 °F/Gas mark 4.*
2 *Heat the oil in a heavy-based pan and sauté the onions for a few minutes until translucent. Add the spices and continue to cook for several minutes.*
3 *Add the beans and tomatoes, bring to the boil, reduce the heat and simmer for 5 minutes.*
4 *Spray a baking dish with oil spray or coat lightly with a little oil.*
5 *Place 3 sheets of lasagne in the bottom, one-quarter of the beans and one-quarter of the cottage cheese. Repeat layers finishing with the beans and cottage cheese.*
6 *Scatter over the mozzarella and bake for 30 minutes until the topping is golden.*

Vegetarian chilli

Vary this classic vegetarian dish with different varieties of beans. Try borlotti beans or flageolet beans for an exciting twist. This chilli provides a good balance of protein, complex carbs, fibre and plenty of vitamins A and C.

MAKES 4 SERVINGS

- 1 tbsp oil
- 1 large onion, chopped
- 2–3 garlic cloves, crushed
- Pinch of chilli powder, according to your taste
- 1 tbsp each of tomato puree and paprika
- 1 400 g (14 oz.) tin chopped tomatoes
- 1 400 g (14 oz.) tin red kidney beans, drained
- 1 400 g (14 oz.) tin cannelini beans, drained
- 500 g (1 lb.) vegetables (e.g. carrots, peppers, courgettes, etc.), chopped

1 *Heat the oil in a large pan. Add the onion, garlic and chilli and sauté for 5 minutes.*
2 *Add the tomato purée and paprika and cook for 2 minutes.*
3 *Add the tinned tomatoes, beans and vegetables. Stir and bring to the boil. Simmer for 20 minutes until the vegetables are tender.*
4 *Serve with cooked rice, pitta bread or crusty bread.*

Bean provencal

Cannelini beans are rich in protein, complex carbohydrates and soluble fibre, which helps to balance blood sugar and insulin levels. The peppers are super-rich in vitamin C, a powerful antioxidant that helps speed recovery after exercise as well as helping to prevent cancer and heart disease.

MAKES 4 SERVINGS

- 1 tbsp olive oil
- 1 onion, sliced
- 1 red pepper, deseeded and sliced
- 1 green pepper, deseeded and sliced
- 1 garlic clove, crushed
- 2 courgettes, trimmed and sliced
- 400 g (14 oz.) tinned chopped tomatoes
- 400 g (14 oz.) tinned cannelini beans or butter beans
- 1 tbsp tomato paste
- 1 tsp dried oregano or basil
- A little low-sodium salt and freshly ground black pepper

1 *Heat the olive oil in a heavy based pan and sauté the onions and peppers over a moderate heat until soft. Add the garlic and courgettes and continue cooking for a further 5 minutes, stirring occasionally.*
2 *Add the tomatoes, beans, tomato paste and dried herbs. Cover and simmer for 15–20 minutes. Season with the low-sodium salt and black pepper.*

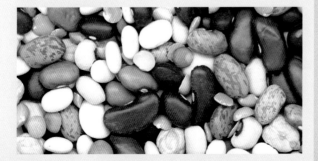

Spicy lentil burgers

These highly nutritious burgers are easy to make and a terrific source of protein, iron and fibre. Accompany with a tomato salsa and Greek yoghurt.

MAKES 4 BURGERS

- 1 tbsp oil
- 1 onion, finely chopped
- 1 tbsp curry powder
- 175 g (6 oz.) red lentils
- 600 ml (1 pt.) vegetable stock
- 125 g (4 oz.) fresh wholemeal breadcrumbs
- Salt and black pepper to taste
- Little oil for brushing
- 4 wholemeal baps
- Salad leaves
- Greek yogurt or tomato salsa

1 *Heat the oil in a large pan and cook the onion until softened. Stir in the curry powder and cook for a further 2 minutes.*
2 *Add the lentils and stock. Bring to the boil and simmer for 20–25 minutes. Alternatively, cook in the pressure cooker for 3 minutes and turn off the heat.*
3 *Allow to cool slightly and mix in the breadcrumbs. Shape into 4 burgers.*
   Place on a lightly oiled baking tray and brush with a little oil.
4 *Bake for 7–10 minutes at 200 °C/400 °F/Gas mark 6 until golden and firm.*
5 *Split the baps and place one burger inside together with salad leaves and a tablespoon of Greek yogurt or tomato salsa.*

Walnut and rosemary burgers

These burgers are really easy to make if you have a food processor. Not only are they super-nutritious, but are also perfect for vegetarian guests at a barbecue. Walnuts are a great source of heart-healthy omega-3 oils, which are important healthy joints and oxygen delivery during exercise. They also supply protein, iron, vitamin E and zinc.

MAKES 8

- 175 g (6 oz.) walnuts
- 140 g (4½ oz.) fresh wholemeal breadcrumbs
- 1 large red onion, finely chopped
- 1 garlic clove, crushed
- 1 tsp dried rosemary
- A little low-sodium salt and freshly ground black pepper
- 2 omega-3 rich eggs

1 Pre-heat the oven to 190°C/375°F/Gas mark 5.
2 Place the walnuts in a food processor and whiz until they are finely ground. 3 Add the breadcrumbs with the onions, garlic, rosemary, low-sodium salt and freshly ground black pepper. Process the mixture for about 30 minutes until it is evenly combined.
4 Add the eggs and process until it holds together firmly. If it is too wet add a few more breadcrumbs.
5 Form the mixture into 8 flat burgers 1.5 cm (¹/₂ in.) thick.
6 Place on an oiled baking tray then brush with olive oil . Bake in the oven for 25–30 minutes until crisp and brown.

Chickpeas with butternut squash

This delicious recipe is one of my favourite winter meals. Chickpeas are an excellent source of fibre, protein and iron. They also contain fructo-oligosaccharides, a type of fibre that maintains healthy gut flora and increases the friendly bacteria of the gut.

MAKES 4 SERVINGS

- 2 tbsp olive oil
- 1 onion, chopped
- 1–2 garlic cloves, crushed
- 1 yellow pepper, chopped
- 1 red pepper, chopped
- ½ butternut squash, peeled and diced
- 1 courgette, trimmed and sliced
- 400 g (14 oz.) tin chopped tomatoes
- 400 g (14 oz.) tin chickpeas, drained and rinsed
- 1 tsp vegetable bouillon powder
- ½ tsp dried thyme
- A handful of fresh basil leaves, chopped

1 Heat the oil in a large heavy-based saucepan and add the onions, garlic and peppers. Cook over a moderate heat for 5 minutes.
2 Add the butternut squash and courgette and continue cooking for a further 5 minutes until the vegetables have softened.
3 Add the tomatoes, chickpeas, vegetable bouillon and thyme. Bring to the boil, and then simmer for 10 minutes.
4 Stir in the fresh basil just before serving with jacket potatoes and extra vegetables.

Roast vegetable lasagne

This tasty vegetarian lasagne can be assembled in less than 30 minutes. It is packed full of protein, complex carbohydrates, fibre, vitamin C, vitamin A and calcium.

MAKES 4 SERVINGS

- ½ large butternut squash, peeled and diced
- ½ red pepper, cut in to strips
- ½ yellow pepper, cut in to strips
- 2 small courgettes, trimmed and thickly sliced
- 1 small red onion, roughly sliced
- ½ aubergine, cut into 2 cm (1 in.) cubes
- 125 g (4 oz.) cherry tomatoes
- A few sprigs of rosemary
- 1 garlic clove, crushed
- 4 tbsp extra virgin olive oil
- 2 × 400 g (14 oz.) tins chopped tomatoes or passata
- 600 ml (1 pt.) cheese sauce (*see* page 164)
- 175 g (6 oz.) lasagne sheets (no pre-cook)

1 *Pre-heat the oven to 200 °C/400 °F/Gas mark 6.*
2 *Place all the vegetables in a large roasting tin. Place the rosemary sprigs between the vegetables and scatter over the crushed garlic. Drizzle with the olive oil.*
3 *Roast in the oven for approximately 30 minutes until the vegetables are slightly charred on the outside and tender in the middle.*
4 *Remove the vegetables from the oven and add the tomatoes or passata, then stir to combine.*
5 *Place a layer of lasagne sheets in a lightly oiled baking dish. Cover with one-third of the vegetable mixture then one-third of the cheese sauce. Continue with the layers, finishing with the cheese sauce.*
6 *Bake for 40–45 minutes.*

Ratatouille with flageolet beans

This dish is super-rich in antioxidant nutrients: vitamin C (from the peppers and green beans), nasuin (from the aubergine), lycopene (from the tomatoes) and quercetin (from the onions). The flageolet beans provide plenty of soluble fibre, protein and iron.

MAKES 4 SERVINGS

- 2 tbsp extra virgin olive oil
- 1 onion, chopped
- 1 each of red, yellow and green peppers, deseeded and sliced
- 2 cloves of garlic, crushed
- 2 courgettes, trimmed and sliced
- 1 aubergine, diced
- 700 g (1½ lb.) tomatoes, skinned and chopped (or use 400 g/14 oz can tomatoes)
- 420 g (15 oz.) tinned flageolet beans, drained
- A little low-sodium salt and freshly ground black pepper
- 2 tbsp basil leaves or chopped fresh parsley

1 *Heat the oil in a large saucepan. Add the chopped onion and peppers and cook gently for 5 minutes.*
2 *Add the garlic, courgettes, aubergines, tomatoes and flageolet beans. Stir then cover and cook over a low heat for 20–25 minutes until all the vegetables are tender.*
3 *Season to taste with low-sodium salt and freshly ground black pepper and stir in the fresh herbs. Serve hot or cold.*

Roasted peppers with rice and goat's cheese

Peppers are packed with vitamin C as well as many other phytonutrients that support the immune system and protect the body from free radical damage. Roasting them in a small quantity of olive oil minimises any destruction of vitamins.

MAKES 4 SERVINGS

- 2 large red peppers
- 3 tbsp extra virgin olive oil
- 1 small onion, chopped
- 2 cloves of garlic, crushed
- 225 g (8 oz.) Basmati rice
- 2 tbsp olive oil
- 1 onion, peeled and chopped
- 2 cloves of garlic, crushed
- 60 g (2 oz.) flaked almonds
- 1 tbsp lemon juice
- 125 g (4 oz.) goat's cheese, roughly sliced
- 2 tbsp chopped fresh coriander

1 *Heat the oven to 190 °C/375 °F/Gas mark 5.*
2 *Cut the peppers in half lengthways, keeping the stalks attached, and remove the seeds. Brush the outsides with a little of the extra virgin olive oil. Place them skin-side down, in a roasting tin, tightly-packed so they do not roll over.*
3 *Bring a large pan of water to the boil. Stir in the Basmati rice. Cover and simmer for 25–30 minutes. Drain.*
4 *Meanwhile, heat the olive oil in a pan, add the onion and garlic and cook over a moderate heat for 5 minutes. Turn up the heat, add the almonds and cook for 1–2 minutes longer, until the nuts are golden.*
5 *Add the onion mixture to the rice, along with the lemon juice, goat's cheese and coriander. Mix together then spoon the rice mixture into the pepper halves.*
6 *Cover the roasting tin tightly with foil and bake for 1 hour until the peppers are tender.*

Tofu and vegetable kebabs with thyme and garlic

These kebabs are a super-tasty and nutritious alternative to the meat version. Tofu is a rich source of protein and calcium and the vegetables provide essential fibre and potassium. Accompany with a tomato salsa.

MAKES 4 SERVINGS

- 250 g (9 oz.) tofu, cut into 16 cubes
- 1 red pepper, halved and deseeded
- 2 small courgettes, each cut into 6 thick slices
- 8 large mushrooms, halved
- 8 cherry tomatoes
- 115 ml (4 fl oz.) extra virgin olive oil
- 2 tbsp chopped fresh thyme
- 1 garlic clove, chopped
- Freshly ground black pepper

1 *Cut the tofu into 16 cubes. Place in a shallow dish.*
2 *Cut the red pepper into 2.5 cm (1 in.) squares. Add to the dish along with the courgettes, mushrooms and tomatoes.*
3 *In a small glass jug, mix together the olive oil, thyme, garlic and freshly ground pepper. Pour over the vegetables. Turn gently to coat. Cover and refrigerate, ideally for 2 hours.*
4 *Thread the tofu and vegetables on skewers, reserving the remaining marinade for basting.*
5 *Cook on the rack of a barbecue or under a hot grill for approximately 8 minutes, turning occasionally and brushing with the reserved marinade.*

Cheese and tomato pizza

MAKES 1 LARGE PIZZA

Base:
- 225 g (8 oz.) strong white flour
- ½ sachet easy blend yeast
- ½ tsp salt
- 175 ml (6 fl oz.) warm water
- 1 tbsp olive oil

Topping:
- 1 tbsp olive oil
- 1 small onion, finely chopped
- 1 garlic clove, crushed
- 300 ml (½ pt.) passata (smooth sieved tomatoes) or 1 400 g (14 oz.) tin chopped tomatoes
- 1 tbsp tomato purée
- 1 tsp dried basil
- ½ tsp sugar
- Pinch of salt and freshly ground black pepper
- 125 g (4 oz.) mozzarella, sliced (or grated Cheddar cheese)

1 *Mix the flour, yeast and salt in a large bowl. Make a well in the centre and add the oil and half of the water. Stir with a wooden spoon, gradually adding more liquid until you have a pliable dough.*
2 *Turn the dough out on to a floured surface and knead for approximately 5 minutes until you have a smooth and elastic dough.*
3 *Place the dough in a clean lightly oiled bowl, cover with a tea-towel and leave in a warm place for approximately 1 hour or until doubled in size (go and have a workout!).*
4 *Knock down the dough, knead briefly before rolling out on a surface to the desired shape.*

5 *Transfer to an oiled pizza dish and finish shaping by hand. The dough should be approximately 5 mm (¹/₄ in.) thick. For a thicker crust, let the dough rise for another 30 minutes.*
6 *For the topping, sauté the onion and garlic in the olive oil for 5 minutes until translucent.*
7 *Add the passata or chopped tomatoes, tomato purée, basil, sugar, salt and pepper. Continue to simmer for 5–10 minutes, or until the sauce has thickened a little.*
8 *Spread the sauce on the pizza base. Scatter over the cheese and any additional toppings from the list below.*
9 *Bake at 220 °C/425 °F/Gas mark 7 for 15–20 minutes.*

Pizza topping ideas:
- Sliced raw vegetables such as tomatoes, mushrooms, peppers, courgettes, asparagus, leeks
- Well-drained cooked spinach
- Sweetcorn
- Thinly sliced tinned artichoke hearts
- Flaked tinned tuna
- Colourful cheeses such as red Leicester or Double Gloucester
- Strong flavoured cheeses such as Parmesan, blue-veined cheese or feta cheese
- Pesto sauce

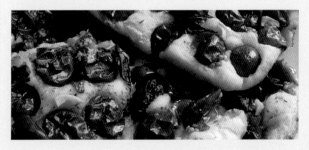

SNACKS AND TREATS

Walnut and date flapjacks

Oats have a low GI and are also a great source of iron, B vitamins and fibre. The walnuts provide omega-3 oils for improved post-workout recovery and heart-health. What better excuse, then, to indulge in these tasty treats?

MAKES 12 FLAPJACKS

- 150 g (5 oz.) butter or margarine
- 60 g (2 oz.) light brown sugar
- 5 tbsp golden syrup
- 200 g (7 oz.) porridge oats
- 60 g (2 oz.) chopped dates
- 100 g (3.5 oz.) chopped walnuts

1 *Pre heat the oven to 180 °C/350 °F/Gas mark 4. Lightly oil a 23 cm (9 in.) square baking tin.*
2 *Put the butter or margarine, sugar and syrup in a heavy-based saucepan and heat together, stirring occasionally, until the butter has melted. Remove from the heat.*
3 *Mix in the oats, dates and walnuts until thoroughly combined.*
4 *Transfer the mixture into the prepared tin, level the surface and bake in the oven for 20–25 minutes until golden brown around the edges but still soft in the middle.*
5 *Leave in the tin to cool. While still warm, score into 12 bars with a sharp knife.*

Muesli bars

MAKES 12 BARS

- 175 g (6 oz.) oats
- 85 g (3 oz.) muesli
- 150 g (5 oz.) dried fruit mixture (e.g. raisins, dates, apricots, figs, apple, pineapple)
- 3 heaped tbsp honey
- 1 egg
- 175 ml (6 fl oz.) apple juice

1 *Combine the oats, muesli and dried fruit in a bowl.*
2 *Warm the honey in a small saucepan until it is runny. Add to the bowl. Stir in the remaining ingredients.*
3 *Press the mixture into a lightly oiled 18 × 28 cm (7 × 11 in.) baking tin. Bake at 180 °C/350 °F/Gas mark 4 for 20–25 minutes until golden. When cool, cut into bars.*

Fruit and nut bars

MAKES 12 BARS

- 60 g (2 oz.) margarine or butter
- 3 heaped tsp honey
- 2 × 125 g (4.5 oz.) cartons plain yogurt
- 225 g (8 oz.) low fat soft cheese or cottage cheese
- 2 eggs
- 60 g (2 oz.) chopped nuts e.g. almonds, walnuts, brazils
- 85 g (3 oz.) sultanas
- 225 g (8 oz.) wholemeal self-raising flour
- 60 ml (2 fl oz.) skimmed milk
- *Optional ingredients:* 25 g (1 oz.) sunflower seeds or pumpkin seeds, 40 g (1.5 oz.) desiccated coconut, 60 g (2 oz.) dried apricots, 60 g (2 oz.) chopped figs

1 *Combine the margarine or butter, honey, yogurt and soft cheese. Beat in the eggs.*
2 *Stir in the remaining ingredients. Add extra milk if mixture seems dry.*
3 *Spoon the mixture into a lightly oiled 18–28 cm (7 × 11 in.) baking tin.*
4 *Bake at 160 °C/325 °F/Gas mark 3 for 35–40 minutes until firm and golden brown. Cut into bars.*

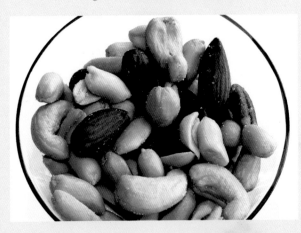

Apricot bars

MAKES 8 BARS

- 125 g (4 oz.) ready-to-eat dried apricots
- 6 tbsp orange juice
- 125 g (4 oz.) self-raising white flour
- 60 g (2 oz.) sugar
- 2 eggs
- 125 g (4 oz.) sultanas

1 *Blend together the apricots and juice in a food processor until smooth.*
2 *Mix together the flour and sugar in a bowl.*
3 *Add the apricot purée, eggs and sultanas. Mix together.*
4 *Spoon the mixture into a 18 cm (7 in.) square cake tin. Bake at 180°C/°F/Gas mark 4 for 30–35 minutes until golden brown. Cut into bars.*

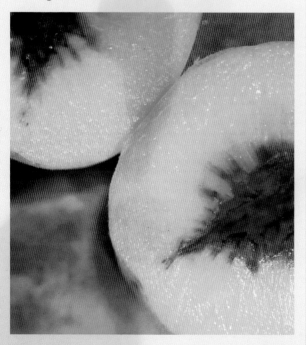

Fruit scones

The secret to making light scones is to mix together the dough very quickly and handle as little as possible. These scones make a nutritious low fat sweet snack, great for refuelling after a workout.

MAKES 10

- 125 g (4 oz.) wholemeal self-raising flour
- 125 g (4 oz.) self-raising white flour
- 1 tsp baking powder
- ¼ tsp salt
- ½ tsp cinnamon
- 60 g (2 oz.) butter
- 40 g (1.5 oz.) sugar
- 175 ml (6 fl oz.) skimmed milk
- 60 g (2 oz.) raisins

1 *In a large bowl, mix together the flours, baking powder, salt and cinnamon.*
2 *Roughly chop the butter and then rub into the flour mixture with your fingertips until it resembles breadcrumbs. Alternatively, mix in a food processor.*
3 *Stir in the sugar.*
4 *Add the milk gradually, mixing quickly with a fork until it forms a soft dough. Do not over mix.*
5 *Press the dough to a thickness of about 1.5 cm (0.5 in.) on a floured surface. Cut into approximately 10 rounds using a scone cutter.*
6 *Transfer onto a lightly oiled baking tray, brush with milk, and bake at 200°C/400°F/Gas mark 6 for 10 minutes until lightly browned on top.*

Oatmeal cookies

These simple cookies are ideal for eating on the move and can be carried in a kit bag/ jersey pocket for a tasty post-workout treat.

MAKES 20 COOKIES

- 4 tbsp margarine or butter
- 75 g (2.5 oz.) brown sugar
- 2 eggs
- 1 tsp vanilla essence
- 150 g (5 oz.) porridge oats
- 85 g (3 oz.) white flour
- ¼ tsp baking powder
- ¼ tsp cinnamon
- 60 g (2 oz.) raisins

1 *Mix together the margarine or butter and sugar until light and fluffy. Beat in the eggs and vanilla.*
2 *Add the remaining ingredients and mix until just combined. You should have a fairly stiff mixture.*
3 *Place spoonfuls on a lightly oiled baking sheet.*
4 *Bake at 180°C/350°F/Gas mark 4 for approximately 10 minutes until golden.*

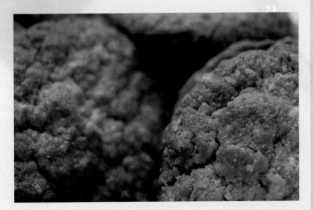

Blueberry and walnut muffins

This recipe is a delicious way of adding antioxidant-rich blueberries to your diet. These muffins are lower in fat than ordinary muffins, providing mostly healthy monounsaturated fats, and richer in fibre and vitamins.

MAKES 12 MUFFINS

- 125 g (4 oz.) self-raising white flour
- 125 g (4 oz.) self-raising wholemeal flour
- 60 g (2 oz.) sugar
- 3 tbsp sunflower oil
- 1 large egg
- 1 tsp vanilla extract
- 200 ml (7 fl oz.) skimmed milk
- 125 g (4 oz.) fresh blueberries or 85 g (3 oz.) dried blueberries
- 60 g (2 oz.) walnut pieces

1 *Pre-heat the oven to 200°C/400°F/Gas mark 6.*
2 *Line 12 muffin tins with paper muffin cases.*
3 *In a bowl, mix together the flours and sugar. In a separate bowl, mix together the oil, egg, apple purée, vanilla and milk then pour into the flour mixture. Stir until just combined.*
4 *Gently fold in the blueberries and walnuts.*
5 *Spoon the mixture into the prepared muffin tins to about two-thirds full and bake for approximately 20 minutes until the muffins are risen and golden.*

Oat apple muffins

Oats provide slow release complex carbohydrate thanks to their soluble fibre content.

MAKES 12 MUFFINS

- 175 g (6 oz.) self-raising flour (white or half wholemeal, half white)
- 125 g (4 oz.) oats
- 125 g (4 oz.) brown sugar
- 2 tsp baking powder
- ½ tsp salt
- 4 tbsp oil
- 1 tsp vanilla essence
- 1 large egg
- 250 ml (8 fl oz.) skimmed milk or buttermilk
- 125 g (4 oz.) grated apples

1 *Mix together the flour, oats, sugar, baking powder and salt in a large bowl.*
2 *Combine the oil, vanilla, egg and milk in a separate bowl then stir into the flour mixture.*
3 *Fold in the fruit.*
4 *Spoon the mixture into lightly oiled muffin tins, filling them two-thirds full.*
5 *Bake in a large bowl at 190 °C/375 °F/Gas mark 5 for approximately 20 minutes until firm to the touch and light brown.*

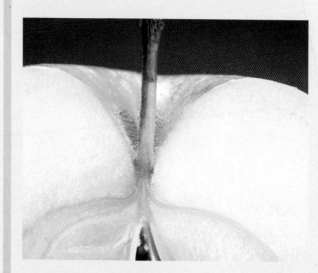

Raisin muffins

The perfect refuelling snack that no athlete should be without! I find that a half and half mixture of white and wholemeal flour gives the lightest result, but you may use just wholemeal flour if you prefer.

MAKES 12 MUFFINS

- 125 g (4 oz.) white self-raising flour
- 125 g (4 oz.) wholemeal self-raising flour
- Pinch of salt
- 40 g (1.5 oz.) soft brown sugar
- 1 tbsp oil
- 1 egg
- 200 ml (7 fl oz.) skimmed milk
- 85 g (3 oz.) raisins

1 *Preheat the oven to 220 °C/425 °F/Gas mark 7.*
2 *Mix the flours and salt together in a bowl. Add the oil, sugar, egg and milk. Mix well.*
3 *Stir in the raisins.*
4 *Spoon into a nonstick muffin tray and bake for approximately 15 minutes until golden brown.*

Chocolate muffins

It is hard to believe that muffins which taste this delicious are fully permitted on a sport diet – but their low fat content makes them quite respectable!

MAKES 12 MUFFINS

- 225 g (8 oz.) self-raising flour (ideally half white, half wholemeal)
- 1 tsp baking powder
- 85 g (3 oz.) sugar
- 40 g (1.5 oz.) cocoa, sieved
- ½ tsp salt
- 2 eggs
- 3 tbsp oil
- 1 tsp vanilla essence
- 300 ml (½ pt.) skimmed milk
- 60 g (2 oz.) chocolate chips

1 *Mix together the flour, baking powder, sugar, cocoa and salt in a large bowl.*
2 *Add the eggs, oil, vanilla and milk and fold together. Add a little extra milk if necessary to produce a very soft mixture.*
3 *Fold in the chocolate.*
4 *Bake at 200 °C/400 °F/Gas mark 6 for 20 minutes.*

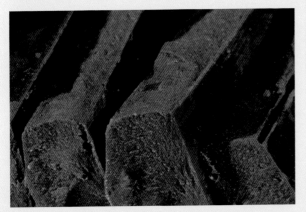

Banana and walnut muffins

These low-fat muffins contain plenty of vitamin B6 (from the bananas), potassium and also omega-3 oils from the walnuts, making them one of the most delicious yet nutritious ways of refuelling after training!

MAKES 12

- 2 large ripe bananas, mashed
- 85 g (3 oz.) sugar
- 60 g (2 oz.) butter
- 1 egg
- 125 ml (4 fl oz.) skimmed milk
- 200 g (7 oz.) self-raising flour
- 60 g (2 oz.) chopped walnuts
- ½ tsp nutmeg

1 *Mix together the bananas, sugar and butter.*
2 *Beat in the egg and milk.*
3 *Fold in the flour, walnuts, salt and nutmeg.*
4 *Spoon into a lightly oiled muffin tin and bake at 190 °C/375 °F/Gas mark 5 for 20 minutes.*

Banana cake

Bursting with vitamins, this fat-free snack could become a staple part of every athlete's diet.

MAKES 12 SLICES

- 2 large ripe bananas
- 250 ml (8 fl oz.) orange juice
- 300 g (10 oz.) self-raising flour (half wholemeal, half white)
- 125 g (4 oz.) brown sugar
- Pinch of salt
- ½ tsp each of mixed spice and cinnamon
- 1 egg
- 1 tbsp oil

1 *Mash the bananas with the orange juice.*
2 *Mix together the flour, sugar, salt and spices in a bowl.*
3 *Add the banana juice mixture together with the egg and oil. Combine together.*
4 *Spoon into a lightly oiled 900 g (2 lb.) loaf tin.*
5 *Bake at 170°C/325°F/Gas mark 4 for about 1 hour. Check the cake is cooked by inserting a skewer or knife into the centre. It should come out clean.*

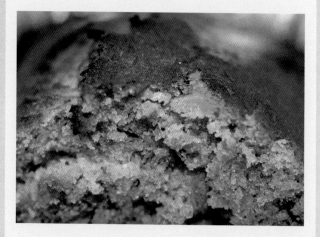

Apple cake

MAKES 12 SLICES

Tasty enough to serve non-athletic guests for tea, as well as refuelling your muscles between workouts, this recipe is a good way of smuggling extra fruit into your diet. It is lower in fat and sugar than conventional cakes and the grated apple and the oil make the cake deliciously moist.

MAKES 12 SLICES

- 300 g (10 oz.) self-raising flour (half wholemeal, half white)
- 125 g (4 oz.) brown sugar
- 1 tsp cinnamon
- 2 cooking apples, peeled and grated
- 4 tbsp sunflower or rapeseed oil
- 2 size 3 eggs
- 125 ml (4 fl oz.) milk

1 *Preheat the oven to 170°C/325°F/Gas mark 4.*
2 *Mix together the flour, sugar and cinnamon in a bowl. Add the grated apple, oil, eggs and milk and combine well.*
3 *Spoon into a lightly oiled loaf tin and bake for about 1–1¼ hours. Check the cake is cooked by inserting a skewer or knife into the centre. It should come out clean.*

Fruit loaf

MAKES 16 SLICES

- 225 g (8 oz.) self-raising flour (half wholemeal, half white)
- 85 g (3 oz.) brown sugar
- 1 tsp cinnamon
- 2 eggs
- 4 tbsp oil
- 1 tsp vanilla
- 225 g (8 oz.) dried fruit mixture (any combination of raisins, sultanas, currants, apricots, dates, pineapple, mango, apple, peaches, figs, papaya)
- 1 apple, grated
- 85 ml (3 fl oz.) skimmed milk

1 *Lightly oil a 900 g (2 lb.) loaf tin. Pre-heat the oven to 180 °C/350 °F/Gas mark 4.*
2 *Mix together the flour, sugar, and cinnamon in a bowl.*
3 *Make a well in the centre and add the eggs, oil, vanilla, fruit and milk. Combine together well.*
4 *Spoon into the prepared tin and bake for approximately 1 hour. Check the cake is cooked by inserting a skewer or knife into the centre. It should come out clean.*
5 *Allow the loaf to cool for 15 minutes in the tin before turning out.*

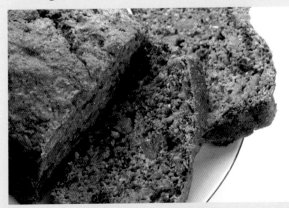

Low-fat chocolate brownies

Traditional brownies are a fat and sugar nightmare. However, my healthier version will allow you to indulge with a clear conscious.

MAKES 16 SQUARES

- 85 g (3 oz.) self-raising white flour
- 40 g (1.5 oz.) cocoa powder
- 175 g (6 oz.) castor sugar
- 125 g (4 fl oz.) vanilla yogurt
- 2 eggs
- 1 tsp vanilla essence
- 1½ tbsp oil
- 25 g (1 oz.) chopped walnuts

1 *Sift the flour and cocoa in a bowl. Add the remaining ingredients and mix together.*
2 *Spoon the mixture into a lightly oiled 20 cm (8 in.) square) baking tin and bake at 180 °C/ 350 °F/Gas mark 4 for approximately 25 minutes until springy to the touch.*
3 *Cool and cut into squares.*

SMOOTHIES

Strawberry and pineapple smoothie

MAKES 2 DRINKS

- 125 g (4 oz.) strawberries, hulled
- ¼ pineapple, cored and chopped
- 125 ml (4 fl oz.) fresh orange juice
- A cupful of crushed ice

Place the ingredients in a smoothie maker, blender or food processor and blend until smooth and frothy. Serve immediately.

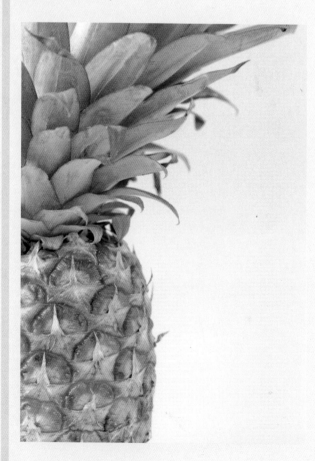

Mango smoothie

MAKES 2 DRINKS

- 4 apricots, stones removed
- ½ mango, peeled, stone removed and chopped
- 1 banana
- 150 ml (5 fl oz.) apple juice
- A large cupful of crushed ice

Place the ingredients in a smoothie maker, blender or food processor and blend until smooth. Serve immediately.

Strawberry and mango smoothie

MAKES 2 DRINKS

- About 12 strawberries
- 1 ripe mango, peeled, stone removed and chopped
- Grated zest and juice of 1 lime
- About 10 ice cubes

Put the strawberries, mango, lime zest and juice and ice cubes in the goblet of a smoothie maker, blender or food processor and process until smooth. Add a little water if you would like a thinner consistency.

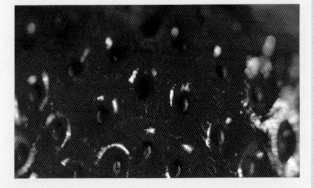

Strawberry and banana smoothie

MAKES 2 DRINKS

- 250 ml (8 fl oz.) orange juice
- 125 g (4 oz.) strawberries
- 2 bananas, frozen and sliced*

Place the orange juice, strawberries and frozen banana slices in a smoothie maker, blender or food processor and process until smooth and thick. Serve immediately.

* Use frozen bananas instead of adding ice cubes to the drinks. Peel bananas, place in a plastic bag and freeze.

Blueberry smoothie

MAKES 2 DRINKS

- 125 g (4 oz.) raspberries
- 125 g (4 oz.) blueberries
- 1 small banana, peeled and cut into chunks
- 125 ml (4 fl oz.) fresh orange juice
- A cupful of crushed ice

Place the ingredients in a smoothie maker, blender food processor and blend until smooth and frothy. Serve immediately.

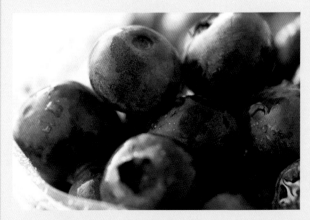

Tropical smoothie

MAKES 2 DRINKS

- About 10 ice cubes
- Juice and zest of 1 lime
- 125 g (4 oz.) strawberries
- 125 g (4 oz.) fresh pineapple
- ½ mango, peeled and roughly chopped
- ¼ Galia melon, peeled and chopped
- 1 banana, peeled and roughly chopped

1 *Place the ice cubes in the goblet of a smoothie maker, blender or food processor and process until slushy.*
2 *Add the remaining ingredients, in batches if necessary, and blend until smooth. Serve in chilled glasses immediately.*

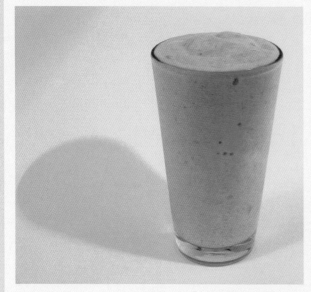

Cranberry smoothie

MAKES 2 DRINKS

- A small cupful of crushed ice
- 250 ml (8 fl oz.) cranberry juice drink
- 60 g (2 oz.) raspberries
- 1 150 g (5 oz.) carton natural yoghurt

Place the ingredients in a smoothie maker, blender or food processor and blend until smooth and frothy. Serve immediately.

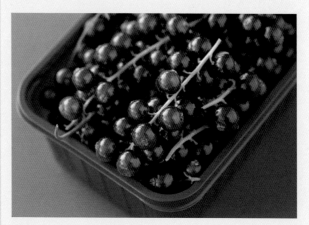

Berry smoothie

MAKES 2 DRINKS

- Approximately 5–6 ice cubes, crushed
- 85 g (3 oz.) strawberries
- 60 g (2 oz.) raspberries
- 1 banana
- 200 ml (7 fl oz.) orange juice

Place the ingredients in a smoothie maker, blender or food processor and blend until smooth and frothy. Serve immediately.

further information

useful addresses

British Dietetic Association
5th floor, Charles House
148–9 Great Charles Street
Queensway
Birmingham, B3 3HT
www.bda.uk.com

British Nutrition Foundation
High Holborn House
52–54 High Holborn
London, WC1V 6RQ
www.nutrition.org.uk/

Dietitians in Sport and Exercise Nutrition (DISEN)
PO Box 22360
London, W13 9FL
www.disen.org/

Eating Disorders Association
1st floor, Wensum House
103 Prince of Wales Road
Norwich, NR1 1DW
www.edauk.com

Food Standards Agency
Room 621, Hannibal House
PO Box 30080
London, SE1 6YA
www.foodstandards.gov.uk

National Sports Medicine Institute of the UK
32 Devonshire Street
London, W1G 6PX
www.nsmi.org.uk

The Nutrition Society
10 Cambridge Court
210 Shepherds Bush Road
London, W6 7NJ
www.nutritionsociety.org/

Vegetarian Society
Parkdale
Dunham Road
Altrincham
Cheshire, WA14 4QG
www.vegsoc.org

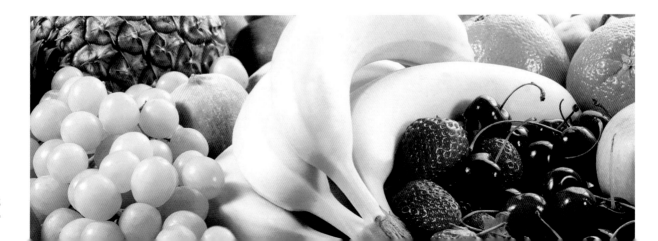

online resources

American Dietetic Association

www.eatright.org

The website of the American Dietetic Association, gives nutrition news, tips and resources.

British Dietetic Association

www.bda.uk.com

The website of the British Dietetic Association includes fact sheets and information on healthy eating for children. It also provides details of Registered Dietitians working in private practice.

British Nutrition Foundation

www.nutrition.org.uk

The website of the British Nutrition Foundation, contains information, fact sheets and educational resources on nutrition and health.

Drug Information Database (DID)

www.didglobal.com

An online service that provides athletes and their support personnel with fast and accurate information about which drugs and other substances are prohibited under the rules of sport.

Eating Disorders Association

www.edauk.com

This website offers information and help on all aspects of eating disorders.

Food Standards Agency

www.eatwell.gov.uk

The website of the government's Food Standards Agency has news of nutrition surveys, nutrition and health information.

Gatorade Sports Science Institute

www.gssiweb.com

This website provides a good database of articles and consensus papers on nutritional topics written by experts.

The Health Supplements Information Service

www.hsis.org

Provides good information on vitamins, minerals and supplements.

Runners World Magazine

www.runnersworld.co.uk

The website of the UK edition of *Runner's World* magazine provides an extensive library of excellent articles on nutrition, training, and sports injuries, and sports nutrition product reviews.

WebMD.com

www.webmd.com

This comprehensive US website has a directory of food topics and advice on many aspects of nutrition and fitness.

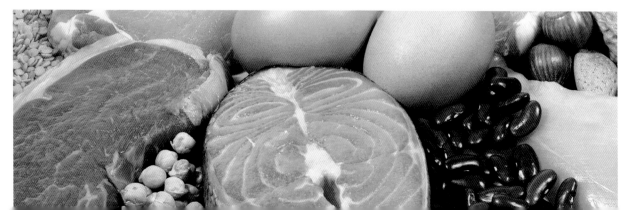

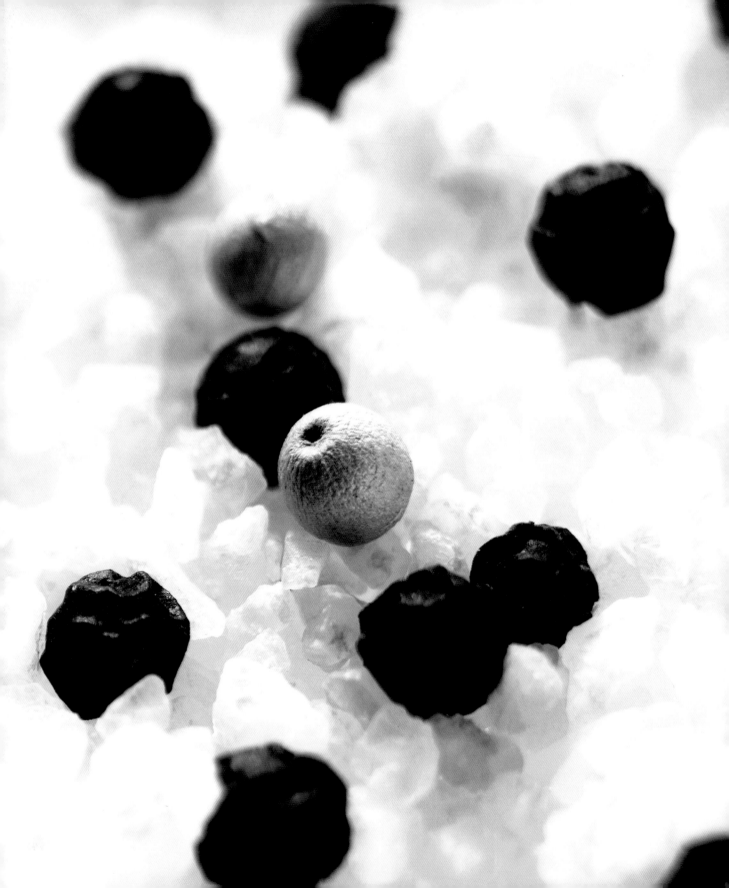

general index

recipe index